DEEP TISSUE SCULPTING

A Technical and Artistic Manual for Therapeutic Bodywork Practitioners

Expanded and Updated Second Edition

Carole Osborne-Sheets
Author of *Pre- and Perinatal Massage Therapy*

Published by
Body Therapy Associates
9449 Balboa Avenue Ste. 310, San Diego, California USA 92123
(858) 277-8827 • (800) 586-8322 • www.bodytherapyassociates.com

Credits
First edition designed by Paradis Design, with typesetting by Sunshine Design and publishing
consultation by Casey Mann Marketing Services. Original photographs by Bill Tutokey
and artwork by Hugo Martines. Published in conjunction with
International Professional School of Bodywork (IPSB), San Diego, California.

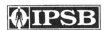

Second edition design and publishing consultation by Sue Bair of Egads.
Additional photography by Andy Sheets,
Jeff Tippet (pp. 10, 60, 108, 119, 127, 133) and Beth Banner (p.107).
Photo models: Donna Seda, Ray Hruby, Andy Sheets, Elizabeth Sheets, Jane Blount and Zach Salazar

Acknowledgements
Rolfing is a servicemark of the Rolf Institute
Arica is a trademark of the Arica Institute, Inc.
Psychocalisthenics, Chua K'a, Domains of Consciousness, Enneagon,
Levels of Consciousness, and Nine Hypergnostic Systems are servicemarks of the Arica Institute Inc.

This book is not intended, nor should it be regarded, as a substitute for the advice of licensed medical professionals. For such advice, readers should consult a licensed physician. Practitioners and clients should refer to the chapters on contraindications and heed all precautions for therapeutic bodywork. If there are health concerns involving illness or injury, medical opinion should be sought. If recipients of bodywork experience serious or protracted pain during or after sculpting sessions, they may have underlying problems that need prompt medical attention. Author, editors, reviewers, and publisher disclaim all responsibility arising from any adverse effects or results that occur or might occur as a result of the inappropriate application of any of the information contained in this book.

ISBN 978-0-9665585-2-4
5 2 8 9 5
9 780966 558524

This book is dedicated
to

Sandy Karst
aka Sara Roundtree

1948 - 1984

My Dear Friend and Midwife to the Rebirth of my Spirit

• • •

Second Edition is dedicated to

Charles Osborne

1921 - 2000

My dear father, and teacher of excellence rather than perfection; he
taught me the futility in worrying, and the joy of both hard work and play.

Contents

Chapter 3
Structural Alignment and the Role of Injury and Illness in Back and Neck Pain . . 33

Chapter 4
Body/Mind: The Role of Emotions in Chronic Tension and Pain 47

Chapter 5
How to Sculpt 57

Chapter 9
Deep Tissue Sculpting Session for the Neck and Shoulders 101

Chapter 10
Full Body Sculpting and Applications to Other Body Areas 111

Tableside Technique Guide

ASSIMILATING

Chapter 11
Integrating Deep Tissue Sculpting into a Practice 117

Chapter 12

SUPPLEMENTING

My Calling

From its earliest stirrings in 1972, my bodywork has been an expression of my heart. Totally in love at the time, I found myself fascinated with my lover, including his bones.

I wanted to know him, and so I explored the depths of his muscles and each bump and curve of his skeleton with an intense curiosity and devotion. I discovered that, when I could feel my way into him, his skin and muscles melted and opened beneath my touch, and I could reach ever deeper inside him.

My fascination quickly spread to every available friend, family member or body that I was with for longer than a few minutes. The similarities and uniqueness of the human body captivated me. I lingered over anatomy texts to identify the territory that was becoming familiar to my pioneering hands. I probed myself for comparisons. It only dawned on me that perhaps I was doing some type of massage when the people who were the objects of my fervor began commenting that they felt relaxed and profoundly known by my touch. Is this what a massage would do, I wondered?

For several years prior, Gestalt and primal reeducation seminars had been part of my training at a center in New Orleans. It was a natural response for me to begin blending deep tissue work with the emotive work of the therapists there. Although by day I taught English and journalism at a public high school, by night, I helped facilitate primal release with my touch. I already knew that I was in my life's work. Finally, the vocation, or calling from God, that I had prayed for so fervently in my devoted Catholic years, had come.

After a year and several disappointing attempts to learn more about this type of massage that I had discovered, I stumbled upon Chua K'a. Teachers from the Arica Institute in New Orleans were teaching this self-massage class. Imagine my reaction when the instructor explained that there was a centuries-old tradition of almost exactly what I had been so obsessively exploring on my own! We touched to the bone our entire bodies, seeking to know ourselves with a newly discovered depth and clarity. We were simultaneously the subjects of an intense anatomy study and the objects of our own most pure, loving and spiritual energy! I continued to participate in the evolution of consciousness trainings of the Arica Institute, including Chua K'a at the Institute headquarters in New York City.

In 1976, I moved to San Diego to pursue my love of the body/mind full time. I studied tai chi chuan with Master Abraham Liu. Within tai chi, I began to employ principles of body mechanics and energy usage that empowered my bodywork. I underwent tremendous change beneath the hands and within the loving energy of psychologist Edward Maupin, Ph.D., my Rolfer. He took me in and became my mentor, teaching me structural techniques to enhance the intuitive, emotive work that was already my skill. Eventually I came to learn the forms with which most practitioners begin, Swedish and Esalen massage, and I pursued my interest in passive joint movement, studying with Dr. Milton Trager, M.D.

When I co-founded a body therapy school in 1977, the Institute of PsychoStructural Balancing (IPSB), now the International Professional School of Bodywork, we coined the name "sculpting" to label the related-yet-different system of deep tissue work that had been synthesized from our various explorations.

Since 1974 I have taught deep tissue sculpting, integrative somatic bodywork, and prenatal body therapy to students in California, around the US and Canada, back home in New Orleans, and even as far from home as Amsterdam. I still feel renewed by the simplicity and the profundity of reaching through the disorder of chronic myofascial tension to touch the human skeleton. I still feel the calling - to know and love others, God, and myself through the body.

For years I thought I wanted to write this book, and it was something I felt I should do. I enviously watched as others published their work. Yet, I never did it. Then, somehow, I relaxed more into enjoying the fruits of the harvest of my life: my family, my home and my garden, IPSB, my practice. Within that celebration there was less urgency to do more, and then I just felt called to write.

Carole Osborne-Sheets

September, 1990

Preface to Second Edition
Called Again

In the twelve years since originally writing this book, much has happened. In life's larger movements, twelve years is but a muscle twitch; from my perspective, though, its been an intricate dance. Broad changes, professional and personal, have challenged and improved my balance and rhythm. Waves of growth have swept therapeutic massage and bodywork into a maturing healthcare practice. The developmental tempo is brisk as schools and jurisdictions implement more rigorous and comprehensive educational standards. Academic and practice-based touch therapy research accumulates, verifying the movement that our hands and our hearts follow daily with each individual client. Even our professional partners have become diverse as massage therapy complements more healthcare providers' practices in a continually broadening variety of settings.

So, I'm called again, for another rendition. Simply put, this revised and expanded edition features the following changes:

- I've included of over another decade's worth of insights. Many of these are my own, gleaned from thousands of sculpting hours with my own clients. Other additions originated from other respected teachers, authors and researchers. Their fine writing and instructional programs, and my dialogues with them and other colleagues add counterpoint and refinement to this edition.

- Expanded content and explanations offer greater clarity, as well as depth and breadth of understanding of the concepts involved in myofascial bodywork.

- Reworked grammar and stylistic modifications help it read and flow more like a friendly classroom environment.

- I've made some rearrangement, both between and within chapters, most notably in Chapters One through Six for greater fluidity and more logical presentation.

- Changes make studying from and referring to this book easier, more effective, and more pleasurably in tune with students' learning needs. Changes include bulleted lists, chapter summaries, more white space, clearer outlines, and other formatting and design details.

- New technique photographs are embedded within the verbal instructions for every technique taught, with graphically enhanced directions on all.

- Musculoskeletal names are standardized for consistency with Andrew Biel's *Trail Guide to Human Anatomy*, from which many schools have adopted anatomy references.

• Horizontally oriented charts outline the three sessions taught, and are printed on heavier stock for easier use and movement at the table during practice.

Upgrading this book has been a creative challenge and pleasure. There's been much to orchestrate to make it happen. I hope the results will serve you and your clients well, and that the rhythm suits you.

Carole Osborne-Sheets
May 2002

Acknowledgements

This book never could have been created or completed without the support and assistance of many. For their many and varied contributions to this book, I thank most deeply:

- My husband, Andy, for his after-hours computer consultations and photography sessions, his dedicated encouragement and perspective in difficult times, and his help in making time and energy available for writing
- My children, Joshua and Elizabeth, for their sharing of my creative and nurturing energies with this other "baby," and for just being themselves; special thanks to Josh for perserverance in refining the Second Edition art and photographs, and to Elizabeth for modeling
- My parents, Shirley and Charles Osborne, for their love, encouragement, and assistance in making the First Edition possible
- My primary teachers, most notably Abraham Liu, Ed Maupin, Ph.D., Ray Hruby, D.O., Milton Trager, M.D., Arica Institute instructors, the late Richard Darby, D.O., of the Upledger Institute, and fellow faculty members at IPSB, especially Diana Panara, James Stewart, Bill Helm, Rick Gold, and Kate Jordan
- My other teachers—the clients and students with whom I have been honored to work since 1974
- The many teachers and practitioners in the bodywork, massage therapy, psychotherapeutic, and manual medicine professions whose writings, work, and teaching have furthered my understanding of somatic therapies
- The somatic practitioners, authors, and teachers whose input to this Second Edition added accuracy, clarity, and wider perspective; particular thanks to Tracy Walton, Tom Myers, Jeff Linn, Diana Panara, June Western, Eugenie Newton, Janis Johnson, Jack Baker, Linda Hickey, and Ron Floyd
- Nancy Ursulak, whose thoughtful, creative, and knowledgeable ideas and editing shaped many of the format changes and reorganizing of material toward a more reader-friendly Second Edition
- My special women friends, who create a circle of support, empathy, and strength around me
- My First Edition editor and longtime friend, Linda Harang, for her sharp pen and wit and for her relentless love for me and my work
- My Second Edition editor, Jeanne Sapp, for her green pens and her crisp, prompt editing
- My publishing consultants, Casey Mann (First Edition), and Sue Bair (Second Edition) for their persistence in keeping me on schedule and on purpose and for their perfectionism
- The administration and owners of IPSB, for their sponsorship of the first edition of this book

UNDERSTANDING

- Perspectives On Deep Tissue Sculpting

- Basic Principles of Deep Tissue Sculpting

- Structural Alignment and the Role of Injury and
  Illness in Back and Neck Pain

- Body/Mind: The Role of Emotions in Chronic Tension and Pain

- How to Sculpt

- Health Maintenance for the Practitioner's Hands and Body

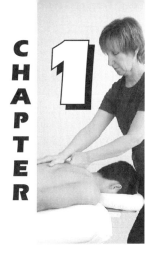

Perspectives On Deep Tissue Sculpting

Why Deep Tissue Sculpting?

Michele's sensitive yet penetrating elbows physically rebalance the athletes who rely on her for pre- and post-event therapy. Rich helps to melt away muscular tension, preparing chiropractic patients for manipulative treatment. Adult children of alcoholics and abuse survivors supplement their psychotherapy with Barbara's focused, empathetic touch. Massage technicians at a world-renowned spa slowly, gently effect lasting tension relief for the guests.

For these practitioners and hundreds of other successful therapists, deep tissue sculpting is one of their most effective, practical techniques for the release of chronic tension. Penetrating, yet nonintrusive, deep tissue sculpting has proven to be reliable in releasing soft tissue tension and pain associated with stress, overexertion, and some injuries and illnesses.

While earning reliable, substantive incomes from satisfied clientele, these practitioners also have avoided the expense of low-back pain, achy joints, and other injuries that many practitioners incur. They have fostered stress-free body mechanics, applying them to all body therapy modalities that they practice. In doing so, they have escaped the overuse syndromes and physical and emotional burnout that plagues others' careers.

Why deep tissue sculpting? It produces effective, lasting relief of chronic muscular tension and soft tissue pain and dysfunction, thereby creating viable practices without harm to the practitioner.

Context

The profession of therapeutic bodywork and massage (somatic therapies) consists of at least the following general methodological categories: circulatory massage, myofascial methods, passive and active movements (performed by or with the practitioner), energy systems balancing, reflexive methods, somato-emotional approaches, and movement and exercise systems (Aston Patterning, Feldenkrais, yoga, etc.).

As a generic category, myofascial work includes sculpting, structural balancing, and self-massage (as taught at the International Professional School of Bodywork, San Diego, California). It also includes Rolfing[sm], Chua K'a[sm], lomi-lomi, Hellerwork, postural integration, myofascial release, trigger point therapy, neuromuscular technique, deep compression massage, and other unique methods of working with the deeper muscles and fascia. Practitioners of other myofascial methods will see consistencies in technique and effect between their work and sculpting as taught in this manual. There are even similarities and crossover effects in such seemingly different work as shiatsu, craniosacral manipulation, and other osteopathic soft tissue techniques.

Soft tissue release has been an integral part of osteopathic manipulative medical care for over 100 years. In the U.S., however, only since 1985 has there been a surging interest in massage therapy, particularly therapeutic methods such as deep tissue work. This was when sports applications of massage for the Olympics and other publicized events began to bring public attention to the emerging massage therapy profession. Several more recent studies, including one conducted by the Stanford Center for Research in Disease Prevention[1] and another reported in the Journal of the *American Medical Association*[2], have documented increased client utilization and favorable physician reactions to massage therapy during the last decade.

Most bodywork practitioners, whether called massage therapist, somatic therapist, massotherapist, holistic healthcare practitioner, or neuromuscular therapist, extensively utilize some myofascial method in their hands-on repertoire. Deep tissue sculpting, specifically, forms the basis of the work of many practitioners in varying settings. They pursue private therapeutic practices and/or work in the offices of or in conjunction with psychologists and counselors, physical therapists, chiropractors, medical doctors, or osteopaths. Indeed, some of these practitioners augment their practices with deep tissue and other soft tissue therapy, i.e. massage therapy.

According to medical historian, Harris Coulter, there are two traditions of medicine, the rational and the empirical. Both are equally grounded in operating principles and historical longevity. In the past century the rational school of health and healing has dominated medical thinking in the Western Hemisphere, and allopathic medicine has reigned supreme. Massage and body therapy are, therefore, commonly understood as "alternative treatments" or, more recently, "complementary." Body therapies are a traditional method of the empirical school of health care, a paradigm with origins in many ancient cultures. Bodywork shares the basic philosophical premises of other empirical methods such as acupuncture and homeopathy. Coulter details the conflict between these two predominant traditions of thought in three volumes, *Divided Legacy*.[3]

The object of the empirical methods is a study of the enhancement and balancing of the "life force" or vital energy. Empirical methods utilize observation and experience as sources of knowledge and view the individual as energetic and having a spiritual dimension. They are holistic methodologies that see health as both an internal and environmental balance. Thus, rather than an "alternative" treatment, deep tissue sculpting and other somatic therapies are viable methodologies for optimal health.

Definition

Sculpting is a form of deep tissue massage characterized by firm, constant compressions and strokes applied parallel to the muscle fibers. Like other myofascial bodywork methods, the techniques are intended to affect the deeper structures of the musculoskeletal system, as well as the skin and the more superficial fascia and muscles. In order to reach these deeper layers, the sculptor uses fingertips, knuckles, elbows, forearms, heels of hand, or any bony body part as tools. Pressure is gradually applied to a tight area until a resistance is met. Constant pressure is maintained while the tissue relaxes and until release is completed, or until the practitioner accepts that no change is forthcoming. The work proceeds slowly to allow the client to assimilate the deeper pressures and the intensity of physical and emotional sensations that can occur. **(Image 1)**

Deep tissue sculpting is partially technical in nature. The methodology has grown from experience and is supported by observation, description, experimental investigations, and theoretical explanations. Yet intuition, emotion, and empathetic connection contribute a vibrant

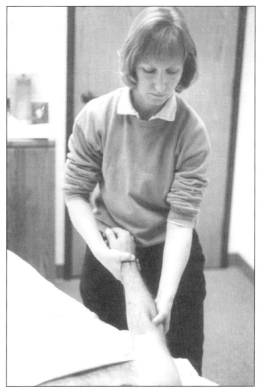

• **Image 1**: *Firm, focused pressure sensitively frees myofascial tissues.*

artistry and holistic dimension to the method. Deep tissue sculpting has a place in our health care system as a sensitive, yet penetrating, method of somatic therapy.

Intentions and Images

The intention of deep tissue sculpting is to create the following effects:
- Organize and restore elasticity to chronically shortened muscle and fascia
- Reestablish independent muscle action
- Open congestion in the muscular attachments to the skeleton
- Increase localized circulation in chronically congested muscles

- Balance intrinsic/extrinsic muscle function and awareness
- Realign posture and movement patterns
- Liberate psychic and emotional tensions held in the myofascia
- Bring consciousness to the core, i.e., the skeleton, by freeing soft tissues of chronic tension

Detailed discussion of these effects follows later in this chapter. (See pp. 14-20.)

The use of the word "sculpting" is deliberately intended to convey the image of the practitioner at work. When doing deep tissue sculpting, the practitioner becomes as a sculpting artist. He figuratively carves away that which is not the essence of the human body, much as the sculptor would remove from a lump of clay or stone that which is not the essence of the object or person he is creating. He holds a mental picture of the muscle or fascial sheath sculpted as it appears in the anatomy books. He imagines the myofascia as free of bunched, constricted, or disorganized areas, and intends his hands to create that.

The practitioner should have a sense of sinking, melting, or soaking into the client's body. Gradual, appropriate levels of pressure and intensity will ensure that tissues are warm. Any pain experienced by the client will feel cleansing and will not produce more tension and resistance. As muscle tension and fascial disorganization melt, the practitioner envisions the skeleton, thereby bringing consciousness to the bone. By imagining the body elongated, the muscles and fascia

lengthened, and space created in the joints, he encourages those very responses.

Indicated Applications

Practitioners find deep tissue sculpting effective with clients who experience the following:

- Generalized tension due to stress or overuse
- Localized chronic muscle tension and myofascial restriction
- Structural misalignments
- Pregnancy-related musculoskeletal discomforts
- Some injuries, diseases, and disorders
- Distorted or diminished body awareness
- Emotional tensions

Localized and generalized myofascial restrictions and misalignments

Deep tissue sculpting is indicated for most forms of chronic muscle tension or fascial restriction, regardless of its cause. It is generally effective with persons who complain of overall body tension due to stress or overuse. It can also produce significant relief in specific areas of chronic tension such as the neck, the low back, or the chest.

It can help individuals with lumbar lordosis, tibial torsion, or other structural misalignments. Structural misalignment is a distortion of the musculoskeletal system. Chronic tension in the muscles, and subsequent binding in fascia, tendons, and ligaments, often restrict the body into inefficient movement patterns and habitual poses and postures. Sculpting techniques can dissolve this tension. For more permanent change, clients need to include movement repatterning and daily stretching.

Pregnancy-related musculoskeletal discomforts

Over half of all expectant women report chronic back pain while pregnant.[4] Many also suffer pelvic, hip, and upper torso pain, often the result of muscle tension, fascial restriction, and postural changes induced by a more anterior center of gravity and an increase in overall body weight. Deep tissue sculpting provides gentle yet deep relief for their tighter postural muscles and strained weight-bearing joints.[5] Many laboring women likewise benefit from the deep pressure of sculpting, depending on the stage of labor and personal preferences. Sculpting practitioners can offer new mothers relief from postural- and mechanical-induced postpartum pain so that they may more comfortably go about their childcare and other activities.[6]

Injuries and diseases

Many accidents and injuries involve associated soft tissue disorders and "splinting" reactions that respond favorably to sculpting. For example, athletes' injured and/or shortened muscles benefit from sculpting, after acute symptoms have resolved and usually on non-event days. Some clients living with autoimmune diseases illnesses, i.e., lupus, scleroderma, or AIDS, or myofascial syndromes such as fibromyalgia also respond well to limited applications of careful, gentle sculpting in conjunction with superficial circulatory techniques.

Sensitive deep tissue sculpting can reduce the shortening of connective tissue and other detrimental effects of conditions of spasticity such as cerebral palsy (CP) and multiple sclerosis (MS). Spasticity is a condition in which certain muscles are continuously contracted causing stiffness or tightness that may interfere with gait, movement, and speech. It may occur in association with spinal cord injury, MS, CP, anoxic brain damage, brain trauma, severe head injury and some metabolic diseases. In these conditions of impaired neurological messaging between muscles and the brain, the respectful awareness of sculpting is especially applicable and effective.

Working closely with and being acutely aware and responsive to the texture/ response of muscle tissue can calm the brain's hypervigilant state. Conversely, bodywork can call attention to or "wake up" hypotonic muscles and tendons. The slow, thoughtful sculpting approach is also conducive to the general neurologically aroused state of individuals with CP or other spastic conditions. Sculpting's slow approach, and firm, solid pressure facilitates relaxation. Sculpting is also predictable movement in that it only occurs with permission of the tissues, so it is very relaxing psychologically and neurologically in and of itself. In chronic conditions, sculpting work is also beneficial in gently and effectively treating the body's reactive or "functional tensions" such as the general strain of seated positions in wheelchairs or walking with crutches.[7]

Altered body awareness and emotional tensions

As a tool for increasing body awareness, sculpting is particularly effective. It goes beneath the client's surface, and its intensity demands that attention be paid to the deeper tissue being worked. Superficial persons and those who tend to be scattered and easily disoriented may benefit from sculpting. This work can deeply touch the overly intellectual person who ignores and disregards her body's messages. It also is useful with many whose body awareness and sense of physical boundaries have been distorted through psychological or physical abuse. Individuals with eating disorders, survivors of sexual abuse, and adult children of alcoholics, for example, often benefit from sculpting, in conjunction with counseling and therapy.[8,9]

Emotional tensions are often the main source of physical tension. The intensity of sensation and a loving, respectful space created by the deep tissue practitioner can create a context for expressing and cleansing emotions. Current stresses and distant psychological trauma melt from the body's soft tissues with a resulting sense of relief and resolution. Many normally functioning people benefit emotionally and physically from this type of expression; however, it is not advisable to pursue deep tissue work with persons with diagnosed or suspected psychopathologies or psychiatric conditions without a qualified therapist's direct supervision.

Of course, consultation with a client's physician concerning most of the above conditions should be a part of the practitioner's approach. Additionally, practitioners and clients should understand that sculpting is not intended to replace appropriate medical care for any condition.

Contraindications

Practitioners should carefully interview and evaluate prospective clients for possible contraindicated conditions, pathologies, or injuries. Medical professionals and many massage therapy authors offer varying lists of these conditions and diseases, often contradicting each other's recommendations.[10, 11, 12] Some of these guidelines are applicable to sculpting; however, the differences in physiological mechanisms between Swedish massage, for example, and sculpting suggest other, more relevant considerations such as those listed below. Emerging information, both from basic science and increasing depth and breadth of clinical massage therapy research, necessitates ongoing modifications to these recommendations. The prudent practitioner will maintain a current knowledge base by ongoing reading and study in the field.

General considerations

Deep tissue practitioners should consider modifying (i.e., lightening pressure, delaying application, omitting areas), being selective in techniques used, or eliminating their sculpting in the following circumstances:

- When clients have any condition that might be spread along the skin (such as impetigo or poison ivy)
- Near or over any wound or area of bone fracture, bleeding (remember that some injuries result in internal bleeding and bruises), skin irritation, discharge, or burns
- In areas of acute inflammation (such

as appendicitis, bursitis, or rheumatoid arthritis), heat, redness, or swelling and pain which are especially vulnerable to deep pressure

- Where clients' tissues are fragile such as on or around bruises and severe varicose veins, over recent surgical sites, or on the extremities of clients with unregulated diabetes

- When a client cannot give reliable feedback on her pain or pressure response due, for example, to numb or anesthetized areas, decreased sensation due to medications, pathology, or alertness state

- When clients have circulatory system disorders such as phlebitis, stroke history, atherosclerosis, and arrhythmias

- With clients diagnosed with fibromyalgia and other chronic myofascial pain[13]

- When clients with undiagnosed lumps, systemic edema, or other undetermined conditions have not yet been evaluated by a physician

- On cancer patients, especially those undergoing radiation, chemotherapy, and other forms of invasive treatment and who often respond better to other forms of massage therapy.[14,15] (Tracy Walton, MS, LMT, who provides advanced instruction for massage therapists working with cancer patients, offers brilliant critical clinical thinking guidelines about cancer and massage therapy. Her insights are particularly useful in evaluating the prudence of deep

tissue sculpting for this specialized population.)[16]

- On individuals presenting injuries or illness that have resulted in muscle strains and tears, sprains, disc injuries, and spinal injuries and with some misalignments and other conditions.[17] (See Chapter Three, pp. 39-44.)

- On clients with discharges, nausea, vomiting, or fever which are symptoms of conditions under which the additional input of prolonged deep tissue work would not be beneficial until resolved

Pre- and perinatal sculpting precautions

While the effects on pregnant women of deep abdominal massage have never been specifically studied, abdominal sculpting is potentially dangerous. Practitioners should maintain a skin and superficial fascial depth on the gravid abdomen.

To avoid legal implications in pregnancy losses, therapists lacking comprehensive training in maternity massage therapy should not work with complicated or high-risk pregnancies, or in the first trimester of all pregnancies. Additionally they should not touch the abdomen in the first trimester and when there is a higher risk of or threatened miscarriage or premature labor.

Other areas of prenatal concern, and in the first 8-10 weeks postpartum, are sites of possible thrombi. These include the veins traversing the inguinal region and the entire medial surface of the legs, specifically along and posterior to the sartorius muscles, distal to the medial knees and along the medial tibial borders.

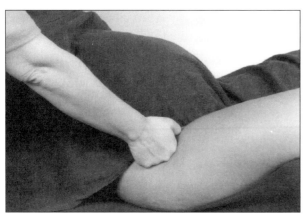

• **Image 2**: *Careful, localized sculpting can reduce prenatal discomforts.*

Sculpting is contraindicated for these areas, as are most other deep, pointed, or jostling techniques. If a client's normal activity level is restricted, further caution is warranted.[18]

If the pregnancy is low-risk and uncomplicated, an expectant woman will usually appreciate appropriate sculpting, especially to other areas of her torso and neck. Care must be taken to avoid increased intrauterine pressure during sculpting, particularly likely when working in the lower back, and when she is prone. Sidelying and semireclining positioning are generally safest and most comfortable throughout most pregnancies. Reflexive points on the feet, lower legs, and back that are sometimes reported to stimulate uterine contractions necessitate broad tools or avoidance when sculpting. Ultimately, it is safest to pursue maternity applications of sculpting and other bodywork only after comprehensive training in pre- and perinatal massage therapy.[19] **(Image 2)**

Endangerment sites

Deep, sustained compression and strokes into some body areas are potentially harmful. These are usually places where blood vessels, nerves or organs are near the body's surface or relatively unprotected. Such commonly identified endangerment sites include: the anterior and posterior neck triangles, the axilla, medial and lateral humeral epicondyles, anterior throat, umbilicus, kidney region, sciatic notch, inguinal triangle, and popliteal fossa.[20] Sculpting in these areas must be slowly, carefully applied, and clients' responses regularly solicited and continually observed. In some cases, sculpting in these locations must be eliminated entirely from a massage therapy routine.

If there is any doubt as to the source of pain and muscle tension that any client presents, or as to the advisability of sculpting for a particular individual, a physician should provide a diagnosis and design treatment plans that advise the practitioner of safety recommendations and precautions.

Tension and its Effect on the Body

Few people escape feeling muscular tension resulting from the stress of everyday life. Pressing commitments to family and friends, driving ambitions, and the struggle to make ends meet all can translate into the body as stiff necks, painful low backs, tight shoulders, or headaches. In addition, most people assume habitual postures and emotions, and then live unconsciously within these prevailing states.

Without appropriate muscle tension,

the body cannot breathe, stand, or walk. Muscular contraction induces breathing by creating air pressure differentials. It holds the body erect, in the field of gravity and moves the body's skeletal structure through space. When muscles contract, tension is produced, but when the muscle is no longer in use the fibers should relax. If this does not happen, a residual tension or contraction remains in the muscle; this residual, excess tension can inhibit the proper functioning of the musculoskeletal system and other body systems. For a more detailed description of the physiological aspects of tension and resulting soft tissue changes, consult the works of Leon Chaitow[21] and Deane Juhan,[22] among other authors.

Tension is not to be confused with tone. Anatomist J.V. Basmajian describes tone as "the state of excitability of the nervous system controlling or influencing skeletal muscle."[23] In an earlier text, he explained that "the general tone of a muscle is determined most by the passive elasticity or turgor of muscular (and fibrous) tissues and by the active (though not continuous) contraction of muscles in response to the reaction of the nervous system to stimuli. Thus, at complete rest, muscle has not lost its tone even though there is no neuromuscular activity in it."[24]

Chronic muscle tension is tension of a prolonged nature, usually gradually increasing in intensity. It can be the result of mechanical strain, environmental factors, physical illness, trauma or injury, emotional trauma, hereditary factors, or physical manifestations of beliefs or ideas of the individual.

Whatever the origin, tension's physiological and mechanical effects are far reaching. Chronic tension:

- Constricts the flow of blood and lymph through vessels and tissues
- Reduces elasticity and shortens the muscle fibers and fascia
- Causes areas of soft tissue to become dysfunctional and intended muscle movements to become disorganized
- Decreases independent and integrated muscular action
- Causes pain
- Can contribute to cardiovascular pathology and hypertension
- Wastes energy
- Interrupts bodily sensation
- Inhibits feelings[25]

In addition, the clinical experiences of many deep tissue practitioners confirm that chronic muscle tension is often accompanied on an emotional level by a corresponding emotional pain, known as a kind of "cellular memory."[26]

Review of Muscular and Connective Tissue Anatomy and Physiology

In order to learn to sculpt, an overview of the construction and functioning of myofascial soft tissues is in order. Not only will the practitioner then be more effective, he will also be more able to explain his use of this modality, its anticipated effects, and his clients' experiences with the work.

General anatomy and physiology

Skeletal muscle (or voluntary, striated muscle) is wrapped in connective tissue

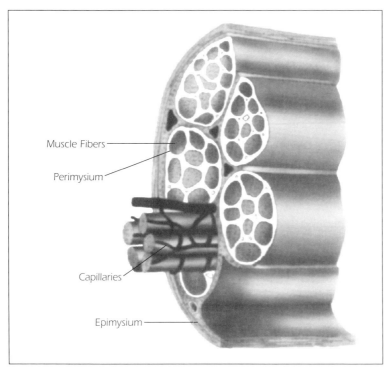

Muscle Fibers

Perimysium

Capillaries

Epimysium

• **Image 3:** *Fascial wrappings intimately invest all layers of skeletal muscle.*

These structures report information to the central nervous system regarding joint position, muscle tone and motion, and speed of activity.

Each muscle cell is enclosed in a delicate membrane, the sarcolemma, which is attached to a fibrous connective tissue surrounding the muscle fiber and separating it from neighboring fibers. Groups of muscle fibers are similarly grouped and separated by coarse fibrous envelopes. Each fiber and fiber bundle is invested with capillaries, arterioles, and venules for blood circulation. An even coarser epimysium encases a whole muscle. The epimysium, also a type of fascial tissue, serves to separate the muscle and its neighbors and permits frictionless movement between them. **(Image 3)**

Groups of muscles are separated into compartments by tough fibrous sheets of connective tissue called intermuscular septa or fascia, which attach to bone and to the investing deep fascia that surrounds all the muscles like bandages. These in turn connect with the superficial fascia just beneath the skin.[27] Muscles and their fascia resemble an orange or grapefruit, with the white, fibrous walls separating and containing the pulp of the fruit. Thus, it is impossible to work with a muscle without

and composed of many bundles of muscle fibers. A muscle fiber is a thread-like arrangement of individual muscle cells. It produces movement because each cell can shorten or contract. The bundled muscle fibers will not contract without stimulus from the nervous system. Each muscle is equipped with a motor nerve that has terminating branches into the muscle fibers. This nerve transmits impulses to the muscle fiber, which normally contracts as a unit to two-thirds to one-half its resting length.

In addition to the motor nerves, there are various sensory reporting organs in and around joints and myofascial tissue, specifically the Ruffin and Golgi end organs, Pacinian corpuscles, muscle spindles, and Golgi tendon receptors.

working with the fascia, the blood vessels, and the nerve network of the muscle.

Fascial components: variations and adaptations

Fascia and the other forms of connective tissue (bones, cartilage, ligaments, tendons, blood, and lymph) all derive from the embryonic mesoderm, and are characterized by large amounts of intercellular material. The various forms of fascia are all constructed of the same materials in differing proportions:

- Specific cells such as fibroblasts, mast cells, and histiocytes
- An amorphous, gelatinous intercellular substance that holds 23 % of the body's water content
- Fibers including collagen, reticular, and elastic fibers which produce the tissue's framework

The specific cells of fascia perform many of the nutritive and defensive functions of the connective tissue system. They participate in phagocytic activity and synthesize antibodies. They also repair tissue injuries by forming scar tissue.[28] This repair activity tends to shorten and make the fascia denser after it heals. These thickened areas will transmit strain in many directions throughout the body, as a pull in a sweater will misshape the entire sweater.[29]

One of the main components of fascia is an amorphous, semifluid interstitial ground substance. This matrix is somewhat of a laboratory[30] in which the other components of connective tissue are both created and perform their activities. It acts as a facilitator and a barrier in the exchange of nutrients and wastes. Its own functions involve important harmonizing dynamics of acid-base equalization, electrical and osmotic balance, and water and salt economy.[31] When the ground substance's supportive functioning is compromised by stress, malnutrition, or other trauma, healthy metabolic activity is disrupted.

The protein and carbohydrate compounds forming connective tissue ground substances vary in their proportions and chemical makeup, creating more viscous gel-like connective tissues in some areas and a more fluid state in others. Ground substances are in a perpetual state of metabolic change, more actively before adulthood, but continuing until death. Ground substance is likely one of the connective tissue components most responsive to the pressure and heat of sculpting and other forms of deep tissue work.

The collagen or white fibers are primarily parallel fibers found together in bundles. The collagen gives tensile strength to the fascia and is densest in ligaments, tendons, and aponeurosis. The elastic or yellow fibers that run singly and branch freely into twisted ropes contribute to its elasticity. The reticular fibers are essentially delicate collagen fibers, and they function to support cells. All of these fibers dry, fray, and become more densely packed as connective tissue ages or is traumatized, playing a role in decreased movement.[32]

Connective tissue ages chronologically and also biologically through injury, illness, and postural and nutritional imbalances. Not only is it denser, but "older" connective tissue is also less fluid, has less elasticity in the collagen, is sometimes accompanied by calcium deposits, has increasing loss of mobility, and recovers more slowly from injury.[33]

Of the different types of fascial layers, the most extensive and the thinnest is the superficial fascia just under the skin. It is the most elastic, and its fibers interlace in all directions. It houses much of the body's fats. It plays a fundamental role in the body's fluid balance, being the mechanism through which the body guides and distributes water.

The deep fascia is denser, but with a smooth coating so that neighboring structures move easily over one another. However, after injury or trauma there is often a gluing effect. Small lumps or bands of thickened, nonresilient tissue can be palpated. Ida Rolf, originator of Structural Integration, explains these lumps as follows:

> They [the lumps] apparently form when the fascial envelope of one muscle attaches itself to a neighboring fascial surface. How this happens is unclear; perhaps the "glue" is a dried exudate secreted in healing a muscle trauma; possibly it results from imperfect healing when a virus has attacked a muscle or tendon. Hans Selye's book, *The Stress of Life*, shows pictures of sacs about the size of walnuts resulting from artificially introducing air into fascial sheaths. Some similarly injurious process no doubt gives rise to the lumpy knotting we have noted.[34]

In a balanced muscle, the connective tissue is perceptibly longer than the muscle fibers that it encloses; however, other areas in the fascia may feel thickened and shortened due to fibrocytic repair activity producing scar tissue or adhesions. In the skin, this cicatricial (scar) tissue first appears quite red with larger blood vessel supply, then gradually whitens as the number of capillaries decreases. The produced cells become smaller and spindle-shaped. This same process of scar tissue formation (cicatrization) occurs even in single muscle cells that have been damaged by inflammations, wounds and necroses.[35]

What Sculpting Does and Why it Works

Liberates and restores elasticity to myofascia and organizes chronically restricted myofascia

Research on connective tissue's mechanical properties substantiates both the lengthening and softening felt under the deep tissue practitioner's hand. Osteopathic research, utilizing the equipment of physicists and engineers, documented the effect of either pressure or traction (load) on connective tissues, including fascia. In these experiments a spring, which is a linear elastic component, represented fascia's elastic and collagen fibers. A small container, called a dashpot, filled with a viscous solution corresponded to the ground substance. Connective tissues like those of muscle and fascia, and to a lesser extent ligaments and tendons, behave like these two components when they are arranged in a series. **(Image 4)**

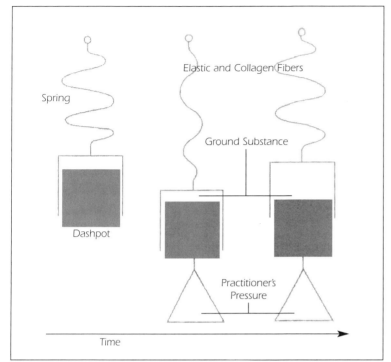

Spring

Elastic and Collagen Fibers

Ground Substance

Dashpot

Practitioner's Pressure

Time

• **Image 4:** *Fascial fibrous and ground substance components respond to pressure over time like a series arrangement of spring and dashpot.*

John Upledger, D.O., explains that when a series arrangement of elastic and collagen fibers (spring) and of ground substance (dashpot) is compressed or tractioned (loaded) the tissue has a characteristic response:

> Load is first accommodated by the stretch of the spring. Then, more slowly, the dashpot begins to move, taking the load off the spring as time passes . . . When the dashpot has totally accommodated the load, and the spring is no longer on stretch, the tissue no longer remembers what it was prior to the deformation imposed by loading ... From this model it is apparent that all dashpots must accommodate all loads imposed in order for permanent corrective change to occur. This movement of the dashpot

requires time. When the spring is no longer under load, the release is palpably perceived by the physician ... There is permanent deformation when the load is removed after sufficient time has passed.[36]

This biomechanical research is applicable not only to sculpting, but probably to all forms of deep tissue work that maintain sustained (ischemic) compressions, such as Rolfing™ and myofascial release. When the practitioner compresses on or tractions the muscle/fascia of a chronically tight area, this touch delivers load to the fascial component arrangement. For best effect, pressure would be sustained evenly at a point of maximum depth without producing resistive effect in the client.

Usually 30 seconds to two minutes of sustained pressure will produce a perceived tissue lengthening or a sinking to a deeper tissue layer. This palpable release is the assumption of the load applied by the practitioner by the fascial ground substance. Sustaining pressure for 10-30 seconds after this sensation helps to ensure a permanent elongation of the connective tissue. The preference for slow, deep pressure recommended here is supported by other properties of fascial tissue: "Viscoelasticity causes it to resist a suddenly applied force but results in gradual elongation to a constantly applied force over time. Creep is the progressive deformation of soft tissues due to constant low loading over time. Hysteresis is the property whereby the work done in deforming a material causes heat and hence energy loss."[37]

Another explanation for the fascia's response to bodywork is its thixotropic quality.[38] Like gelatin, connective tissue solidifies when it sits undisturbed, and it becomes more fluid, seeming to melt when it is stirred up. Connective tissue is "disturbed" by metabolic activity, physical work, aerobic exercise, and stretching. The movement, pressure, friction, thermodynamic heat transfer, and vibratory rhythms of therapeutic bodywork procedures, including deep tissue sculpting, mechanically stimulate fascial energy levels. This results in a more fluid ground substance that conducts more exchanges of nutrients and cellular wastes through the hollow tubes in the collagen fibrils that form the structural framework of the connective tissue.[39]

Ida Rolf explains the biomechanical properties of connective tissue as applied to Rolfing:

> While fascia is characteristically a tissue of collagen fibers, these must be visualized as embedded in ground substance. For the most part, the latter is an amorphous semifluid gel. The collagen fibers are demonstrably slow to change and are a definite chemical entity. Therefore, the speed so clearly apparent in fascial change must be a property of its complex ground substance. The universal distribution of connective tissue calls attention to the likelihood that this colloidal gel is the universal internal environment. Every living cell seems to be in contact with it, and its modification under changes of pressure would account for the wide spectrum of effects seen in Structural Integration.[40]

When pressure is applied parallel to muscle fibers in either a sculpting stroke or compression technique, it exerts a force on the muscle and its fascia. Long-lasting pull elongates the connective tissue system in the direction of the pull.[41] Just as stretching a too-tight garment allows the torso within to stretch and relax more freely, elongation of the fascia permits length and increased elasticity for the formerly shortened, constricted muscle fibers.

Rolfer and anatomy instructor Tom Myers articulates this effect slightly differently, but agrees that it is anything but localized. He sees the myofascia as a collagenous network that connects, wraps, and supports the skeleton. He describes lengthening manipulations of any segment of these myofascial continuities, or myofascial meridians, as ripple-like, universal, and integrative in their effect.[42]

With nonproductive fascial pull alleviated in muscle/tendon units, the sensory organs (muscle spindles and Golgi tendon organs) respond, causing the entire muscle to relax. This reflex relaxation is the usual result of bodywork techniques that involve sustained pressure applied directly to the belly of a contracted muscle or to nearby dysfunctional soft tissue.[43]

Jim Oschman, Ph. D., an academic scientist, has published many articles focused on the scientific basis for various complementary or alternative medicines. He describes connective tissues' cellular structure, physiology, and systemic dynamics, offering further explanation of the changes felt by bodywork practitioners.[44] Physical therapists, John and Mark Barnes' writings synthesize connective tissue changes during myofascial release and emerging theories of information transfer and cellular biology.[45]

Reestablishes independent muscle action and frees congestion in the muscular attachments to the skeleton

When an area is slowly sculpted, muscle fibers that had bunched, shortened, formed adhesions, and become disorganized become elongated and begin functioning in more efficient lines of contracting muscle. The fascia no longer traps and restricts the muscles from elongating. It also no longer serves as a "glue" that attaches neighboring, but differently functioning, muscle groups. Independent functioning of muscles is now possible. For example, the neighboring quadriceps and the adductors often are forced to work together in walking. This is not because the adductors are needed for normal gait, but because confusion and congestion in the fascia that, in effect, tie the two muscle groups together.

Other areas where inappropriate "gluing" by congested fascia occurs are at muscle attachments to bone, particularly broader attachments, such as the tibialis anterior along the shaft of the tibia. With deep tissue sculpting, sites where muscle connects to bone become clearer of scar tissue and residues of metabolic wasteproduct build-up.

Increases localized circulation in chronically congested muscles

Muscles work by nerve stimulation producing contraction of the elastic fibers of the muscle. When a muscle contracts, it burns a type of food called muscle glycogen, which is supplied by the blood and lymph circulation and stored in the muscle for its use. When muscle glycogen burns, it breaks down into a chemical called pyruvate. When enough oxygen is available, pyruvate converts to carbon dioxide and water, which are expelled from the lungs; however, pyruvate converts to lactic acid when the oxygen supply is insufficient. The muscle's ability to respond is diminished when lactic acid builds up in the muscle, producing a state called acidosis.[46]

When a muscle is chronically tight, it does not relax fully after a contraction. Restriction of blood and lymph flow results since movement through the capillaries and interstitial spaces is decreased. When circulation is restricted, acidosis is not relieved, nor is a full capacity supply of nutrients and oxygen possible. A vicious cycle of lactic acid and other wasteproduct build-up and nutritional deficits begins. Pain also develops as both pressure and the muscle's acidic state irritate sensory nerve endings.[47]

When firm, constant pressure is applied to a chronically contracted muscle and then released, the localized effect on circulation may be like the effect of crimping and then releasing a running hose. The released pressure of the blood and lymph serves to power through constricted vessels and tissue, thereby opening and clearing that tissue with the increased flow. A warm, flushed feeling, and sometimes tingling or vibratory sensations, results. This sensation also could be result of the increase in blood flow created by vasomotor response to sculpting pressure.

This is a likely model of the mechanisms involved in sculpting. The elongating effect on the elastic and collagen fibers of the muscle's connective tissue also allows more circulation through the vessels and interstitial spaces of the muscles. Undernourished, brittle fascia becomes nourished and recovers its fluid nature. Thus, recovery from acidosis is facilitated.

The specialized connective tissue that surrounds nerve fibers would appear to also benefit from sculpting manipulations, in turn improving the function of the neurons that they surround and support. In *Job's Body*, Deane Juhan describes these neurons as actually more like tiny glands than the commonly held conception of them as sparking wires; neurotransmitters and a liquid solution of sodium ions transmit information between neurons. Thus, improved circulation of fluids promotes the metabolic functioning of nerves. This may help to clear sensation and thinking, improve muscular precision and responsiveness, and balance sensory thresholds.[48]

In styles of massage that produce generalized increase in circulation, movements always proceed in the direction of blood flow towards the heart. In the case of deep tissue sculpting, however, most of the circulatory effect is localized; therefore, it is not critical that sculpting always be done in the direction of the heart. If any weakness in the vessels of the legs is evident, more superficially sculpting and moving distal to proximal are reasonable precautions. In more severe cases of varicose veins, sculpting the legs is best completely avoided. On the other hand, many clients need to feel the muscles of their extremities elongate toward the feet and hands. Sculpting in the proximal-to-distal direction more readily produces that sensation and could be safe if back pressure is not created in the compromised veins.

Balances intrinsic and extrinsic muscle function and awareness

Extrinsic muscles are the more superficial muscles, such as the biceps brachii and the hamstring group. Being larger and more powerful, they are mostly the muscles of "doing." The extrinsic muscles convey the energy of the outer world into the inner reality of the individual, and vice versa. They are usually under more conscious control than the intrinsic muscles.

The intrinsic muscles are smaller, deeply located muscles that are mostly "being" muscles. These muscles are involved in fine adjustments in posture, balance, and movement. Relay of the internal feelings of the body to the outer muscles for expression to the external world occurs through these muscles. In many individuals the intrinsic muscles, such as the psoas major and the suboccipitals, are not readily available for deliberate, conscious control.[49]

Balance between "doing" and "being," the extrinsic and intrinsic, male and female, and between outer and inner reality is the process of human existence. When the contraction and spasm of chronically tight muscles are released, a more balanced muscular consciousness is possible. The intrinsics can become more available and controllable for their functions, which often have been assumed by the larger extrinsics. The individual then lives more from her inner core and in a more meaningful response to the world outside the self.[50]

Realigns posture and movement patterns

The natural lines of stress-free alignment of the skeleton are more possible when the musculature and the fascia are elongated, elastic, and more conscious. The tensional force of the connective tissue framework, an example of what Buckminster Fuller called "tensegrity," allows for the appropriate spacing of the bones in its matrix.[51] Tensegrity is what makes bipolar extension of the spine possible. Organization of movement within this vertical polarity and around the horizontal planes of the atlas, the pectoral girdle, the pelvis, and the legs is achievable after sculpting. Graceful, balanced movement becomes more apparent.

Long lasting structural change occurs through appropriate hands-on release,

reeducation of movement patterns, and balanced tone/stretch in paired-function muscles, such as the rhomboids and the pectoralis muscles. While deep tissue sculpting changes postural alignment and movement patterns, these goals are usually more precisely addressed with hands-on techniques that first hold tissues in place with sculpting-type compression and then ask for active client movement. (See pp.128-131 for more details on this approach.) Sculpting, accompanied by appropriate stretch and tone exercise and movement repatterning, is also more effective than sculpting alone when structural change is the primary goal. Judith Aston, Thomas Hanna, and F.M. Alexander, among others, have each developed elegant, unique movement education systems for these purposes.

Liberates psychic and emotional tensions held in the myofascia

A wide range of professionals embrace the concept that the body reflects the emotional states of the individual. These professionals include, among others, scientists Candace Pert and James Oschman, and psychologist Peter Levine, psychiatrist Wilhelm Reich, physicians Andrew Weil and Rene Cailliet, and Ida Rolf. Ancient traditions such as Chinese and Ayurvedic medicine, yoga disciplines, and Chua K'a as taught by the Arica Institute, agree. If the corporal body is a reflection of the other "bodies"— emotional, spiritual, and astral—then an intervention such as deep tissue sculpting, which facilitates an opening, elongating, and softening of the soft tissues, will have a corresponding effect on the other noncorporal "bodies."[52]

On the feeling level of the client's experience, emotional release may coincide with myofascial release. Recall of painful and traumatic experiences from even the distant past can occur. Sculpting sometimes elicits intense crying, screaming, kicking, and other expressions of anger, sadness, or fear. Simple yet profound sighs or subtle changes in breathing patterns also may signal the release of a chronically constricted emotion. (See Chapter Four, pp. 47-56.)

Brings consciousness to the skeleton by freeing muscles of chronic tension

With painful, constricting musculature relieved, an individual's awareness can shift from the musculature that is primarily more superficial to the more profound, deeper structures of the bones themselves. The individual's kinesthetic sense of self can thus be increased; rather than a sack of skin and muscles, she becomes a sculpture of bones moving through space and time. Perhaps this shift also translates on a spiritual level to more awareness of one's deeper, truer, God-like Self.

Summary of Chapter One

1. Deep tissue sculpting is one method within the myofascial category of somatic therapies which are, in turn, part of the empirical, holistic approach to healing.
2. Deep tissue sculpting is a form of deep tissue massage characterized by firm, constant compressions and strokes applied parallel to the muscle fibers for the purpose of affecting the deeper structures of the musculoskeletal system, as well as the skin and the more superficial fascia and muscles.
3. By using clear images that guide his method of work and the desired outcomes, the practitioner's work will affect all levels of the client's musculoskeletal system and bring awareness to the psychic and emotional tensions held there.
4. Deep tissue sculpting is indicated for most forms of chronic muscle tension or fascial restriction, regardless of its cause.
5. Deep tissue sculpting provides gentle yet deep relief for women during pregnancy, labor and birth, and postpartum.
6. Some illnesses and injuries involving soft tissue disorders and "splinting" reactions respond favorably to sculpting.
7. Because deep tissue sculpting focuses on the body's deeper tissues, it can clarify a client's body awareness, physical boundaries, and the sources of physical and emotional tensions.
8. Prospective clients should be screened for contraindications standard to all body therapies, as well as for those specific to deep tissue sculpting. Techniques should then be modified or even eliminated. If in doubt about the advisability of sculpting, a physician should diagnose the client and design a treatment plan.
9. It is outside the scope of bodywork and massage therapy practice to diagnose injury or disease.

10. While it is possible to do sculpting and other bodywork on most pregnant women, it is safest to proceed only after comprehensive training in pre- and perinatal massage therapy.

11. Deep, sustained compression and strokes into some body areas are potentially harmful. Sculpting in these areas, if done at all, must be slowly and carefully applied.

12. Chronic muscular tension resulting from the stress of everyday life expresses itself not only as physical pain and discomfort, but also as emotional distress, postural misalignment, loss of vitality and function, and even eventual pathology.

13. Because of the intricate makeup of muscle tissue and fascia and their interrelationship with nerves, blood, and bones, it is impossible to work with a muscle without also working with fascia, the blood vessels, and the nerve network of that muscle.

14. As one kind of connective tissue, fascia occurs in various forms throughout the body, performing many nutritive, balancing, protective and healing functions.

15. Fascia consists of ground substance and collagen, elastic, and reticular fibers. These components change in response to activity level, aging, injury, disease, stress, and therapeutic bodywork techniques.

16. Biomechanically, the practitioner's sustained compression into a chronically tight area loads the ground substance of the fascia and stimulates its energy levels, thus promoting an eventual release of the elastic and collagen fibers of the fascia.

17. Application of long lasting pull elongates the connective tissue system in the direction of the pull, and also allows muscle fibers to lengthen and operate in more efficient lines of contracting muscle.

18. Released fascia that surround neighboring muscles are no longer glued to one another, allowing each muscle to act freely of the other.

19. Scar tissue and wasteproducts where muscle meets bone decrease when congested fascia is unglued at these sites.

20. The elongating effect of the elastic and collagen fibers of the muscle's connective tissue allows more circulation of blood and lymph through the vessels and the interstitial spaces of the muscles. A similar effect is produced around neurons when their connective tissue is lengthened.

21. Balancing the intrinsic/"being" and the extrinsic/"doing" muscle functions and awareness can help individuals balance other aspects of their lives beyond the physical.

22. The natural lines of stress-free alignment of the skeleton are more achievable when the musculature and the fascia are elongated, elastic, and more conscious.

23. Given that the corporal body is a reflection of the "bodies," an intervention that facilitates opening, elongating and softening of the soft tissues will have a corresponding effect on those other "bodies."

24. Freed from chronic muscular tension, an individual can develop a clearer kinesthetic sense of her deepest physical structure – her bones – and perhaps a clearer sense of her spiritual self.

Sources Cited

[1] Stanford University School of Medicine, "Complementary and Alternative Medicine: Scientific Evidence and Steps Towards Integration." Conference held September, 1999.

[2] Eisenberg, et. al. "Trends in Alternative Medicine Use in the United States, 1990-1997." *Journal of the American Medical Association*, 280(18): November 11, 1998, pp.1569-1575.

[3] Coulter, Harris L. "Divided Legacy: The Conflict Between Homeopathy and the American Medical Association." *Science and Ethics in American Medicine*, 1800-1914, Volume III. Richmond, CA: North Atlantic Books, 1982, pp.vii-xii.

[4] Ostgaard, H.C., Andersson, G.B.S., et al. "Prevalence of back pain in pregnancy." *Spine*, January 1992, 17(1), pp.53-55.

[5] Osborne-Sheets, Carole. *Pre- and Perinatal Massage Therapy*. San Diego, CA: Body Therapy Associates, 1999, p.83.

[6] Ibid, p.142.

[7] For more information on working with clients with physical disabilities, contact Linda Hickey, RMT: Synergea Family Health Centre, #9 Arbor Lake Drive N.W., Calgary, Alberta, Canada T3G 5G8. 403-247-2947. maternitymassage@shaw.com

[8] Timms, Robert, Ph.D., Connors, Patrick, C.M.T. *Embodying Healing*. Orwell, VT: Safer Society Press, 1992, pp.48-51.

[9] Carver, Claudia. "Sensitive Treatment for Survivors of Childhood Sexual Abuse." *Massage Magazine*, Jan/Feb, 2001, pp.171-178.

[10] Tappan, Frances M. *Healing Massage Techniques: Holistic, Classic, and Emerging Methods*. USA: Appleton and Lange, 1988, pp.18-20.

[11] Fritz, Sandy. *Mosby's Fundamentals of Therapeutic Massage*. St. Louis, MO: Mosby-Year Book, Inc., 1995, pp.88-101.

[12] Premkumar, Kalyani. *Pathology A to Z: a Handbook for Massage Therapists*. Calgary, AB, Canada: VanPub Books, 1996.

[13] Starlanyl, Devin, M.D. and Mary Ellen Copeland, M.S., M.A. *Fibromyalgia and Chronic Myofascial Pain Syndrome*. Oakland, CA: New Harbinger Publications, Inc., 1996.

[14] Curties, Debra, *R.M.T. Massage Therapy and Cancer*. New Brunswick, Canada: Curties-Overzet Publications, Inc., 1999, pp.36-37.

[15] MacDonald, Gayle. *Medicine Hands: Massage Therapy for People With Cancer*. Forres, Scotland: Findhorn Press, 1999, p.19.

[16] Walton, Tracy. "Clinical Thinking and Cancer." *Massage Therapy Journal*, Fall, 2000, 39: 3, pp.66-80. For training in caring for clients with cancer, contact: Tracy Walton, 10 Sargent Street, Cambridge, MA 02140. 617-576-1300 x3019. Tracywalton@msn.com

[17] Benjamin, Ben E. *Listen to Your Pain*. New York, NY: Penguin Books, 1984, p.33.

[18] Osborne-Sheets, Op. Cit., pp.36-40.

[19] For Pre-and Perinatal Massage Therapy Certification workshops designed by Carole Osborne-Sheets, contact Body Therapy Associates, 11650 Iberia Place, Suite 137, San Diego, CA 92128, 858-748-8827 or 800-586-8322. www.bodytherapyassociates.com

[20] Fritz, Op. Cit., p.97.

[21] Chaitow, Leon. *Modern Neuromuscular Techniques.* New York, NY: Pearson Professional Limited, 1996, pp.1-12.

[22] Juhan, Deane. *Job's Body: A Handbook for Bodywork.* Barrytown, NY: Barrytown Limited, 1998, pp.115-144.

[23] Basmajian, John V., M.D. *Primary Anatomy.* Baltimore, MD: The Williams and Wilkins Co, 1970, p.126.

[24] Basmajian, John V., M.D. *Muscles Alive.* Baltimore, MD: The Williams and Wilkins Co, 1967, p.71.

[25] Chaitow, Op. Cit. p.8.

[26] Drury, Nevill. *The Bodywork Book.* Dorset, England: Prism Alpha, 1984, pp.121-123.

[27] Basmajian, *Primary Anatomy*, Op. Cit., pp.118-121.

[28] Cailliet, Rene, M.D. *Soft Tissue Pain and Disability.* Philadelphia, PA: F.A. Davis Co., 1977, pp.4-8.

[29] Rolf, Ida, Ph.D. *Rolfing: The Integration of Human Structures.* New York, NY: Harper and Row, 1977, p.39.

[30] Snyder, George E, Ph.D. "Fasciae-Applied Anatomy and Physiology". *Journal of the American Osteopathic Association,* March, 1969, 68: pp.675-685.

[31] Dicke, E., H. Schliack, A. Wolff. *A Manual of Reflexive Therapy of the Connective Tissue (Connective Tissue Massage) "Bindegewebsmassage".* Scarsdale, NY: Sidney S. Simon, 1978, p.44.

[32] Cailliet, Op. Cit., p.6.

[33] Rolf, Op, Cit., p.184.

[34] Rolf, Op. Cit., p.129.

[35] Dicke, Op. Cit., p.45.

[36] Upledger, John E., D.O., and Jon D. Vredevoogd, D.O. *Craniosacral Therapy.* Seattle, WA: Eastland Press, 1983, p.130.

[37] Twomley L., J. Taylor. "Flexion, Creep, Dysfunction and Hysteresis in the Lumbar Vertebral Column," S*pine,* 1982: 7,2, pp.116-122.

[38] Juhan, Op. Cit., p.68.

[39] Juhan, Op. Cit., p.69.

[40] Rolf, Op. Cit., pp.41-42.

[41] Dicke, Op. Cit., p.45.

[42] Myers, Tom. *The Anatomy Trains: Myofascial Meridians for Manual and Movement Therapists.* Edinburgh, UK: Churchill Livingstone, 2001.

[43] Chaitow, Op. Cit., p.37.

[44] Oschman, Jim. "What is Healing Energy? Part 5: gravity, structure, and emotions." *Journal of Bodywork and Movement Therapies,* October, 1997, pp.297-309.

[45] Barnes, Mark F, MPT. "The Basic Science of Myofascial Release: Morphologic change in connective tissue." *Journal of Bodywork and Movement Therapies,* July 1997, pp. 231-238.

[46] Juhan, Op. Cit., pp.123-133.

[47] Chaitow, Op. Cit., p.23.

[48] Juhan, Op. Cit., pp.157-158.

[49] Maupin, Edward W., Ph.D. *The Structural Metaphor* (Part one). San Diego, CA: International Professional School of Bodywork, 2001, p.30.

[50] Drury, Op. Cit., p.120.

[51] Juhan, Op. Cit., p.82.

[52] Maupin, Edward W., Ph. D. *The Genie in the Bottle: Psychology for Bodyworkers.* San Diego, CA: International Professional School of Bodywork, 1992, pp. 1-17.

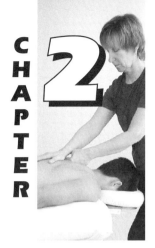

CHAPTER 2

Basic Principles of Deep Tissue Sculpting

Before moving into how and where for specific sculpting techniques, understanding the underlying principles of the method is useful. Principles state the assumptions, operating beliefs, and the laws or rules determining characteristic behaviors and outcomes of a system. These are not necessarily proven truths, but they are the assumptions and paradigms that appear to be operating while sculpting and interacting with a body therapy client. Principles can provide hypotheses worthy of further investigation. Practice observation, case studies, and other research methodologies create varying levels of verification of the veracity of these principles. This chapter includes principles of conscious bodywork, which sculpting certainly is intended to be. Discussion of the specific underlying processes involved in sculpting completes this chapter.

Principles of Conscious Bodywork

Edward Maupin, psychologist and one of the first seven students of Ida Rolf's system of structural integration, teaches one of the simplest, yet most encompassing, expositions of bodywork's basic principles. These concepts are described below as he first articulated them, and further expansions on these principles can be found in his publications, including *The Structural Metaphor.*[1]

1. Technique follows perception.
2. Perception is a function of love.
3. What you imagine or visualize is what you will touch or create.
4. The balance of receptive and active energies is the process of bodywork.

Technique follows perception

When the practitioner approaches a client, she must evaluate this individual at that moment. Then she makes decisions as to what type of work is appropriate and what specific techniques from a particular method are to be used. If she first tunes into the client and observes with all senses, she can more fully utilize her receptive faculties. Tuning in includes her sensory observations, augmented by information and impressions gleaned from their interactions, and by her intuition. She must approach her client with the simple, receptive energy of "knowing" her client rather than "fixing" him. When action does come forth, it is likely to be more responsive to the client's needs. The work is then more effective than if she either uses a routine or whatever she happens to do best or most easily.

Perception is a function of love

The Latin root for "perception" means *to seize wholly.* By engaging not only her senses but also her intuition and the physical, emotional, and intellectual powers, the practitioner can develop a more complete understanding of her client. This principle emphasizes the role that Love, without ego and in its most universal state, plays in perception. When a practitioner observes her client with Love, then there is a recognition that the Spirits of the client and her own are as One. There is a sense of empathy with all aspects of the individual. There is respect, equality, and appropriate responsibility.

What you imagine or visualize is what you will touch or create

There are many possible goals in bodywork. These include:

- Physical healing
- Structural organization
- Enhanced sensory awareness
- Organization of energy
- Emotional release
- Recovery of traumatic memory
- Therapeutic intimacy[2]

The body also has many levels that a practitioner can touch, including the skin and fat, the external fascia, the muscles, the bones, and the energy flows. Of course, within these goals and these levels the practitioner can focus on many specific effects and structures. Whatever she thinks, imagines, visualizes, or focuses on is where she will touch; this determines what effect will be created, respecting the factor of the client's readiness to receive and respond. This principle acknowledges the result of focus or intention in effective body therapy. It also reminds the practitioner that unclear intention, absentminded routines, and general clutter and chatter in the mind will interfere in a most defeating way with the goals of conscious bodywork.

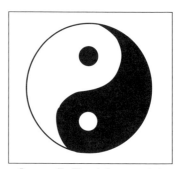

- **Image 5:** *The yin/yang symbol conveys balance of opposites.*

The balance of receptive and active energies is the process of bodywork

Natural, effortless movement between receptive and active energy is the overall goal of many forms of body therapy. The receptive (yin) energy is attractive, open-ended, nongoal-oriented, omnidirectional, and artistic. The active (yang) energy is more goal-oriented, linear, and directed. The traditional Oriental symbol depicts this balancing process as a circle with the yin half black, and the yang half white. Within each lies a seed of the other.[3]

(Image 5)

On a more anatomical and functional level, brain activity in the cerebral hemispheres reflects this balance of energies. Analytical, logical thinking, especially as used in verbal and mathematical function, involves more of the left hemisphere. The right hemisphere handles space, creativity, body image, and other non-linear thought processes. Interestingly enough, as further evidence of the balance of these seeming opposites, the left cerebral hemisphere controls most of the right side of the body's motor and neuromuscular functions, and the right orchestrates the same activities for the left side.[4]

A balance of active/receptive and left/right brain functions within the practitioner is crucial. As she interacts with her client, she must cultivate active receptivity. In other words, the practitioner looks to her perception to guide her actions. She allows the client to respond and open to her touch rather than force technique on the client. The practitioner visualizes and focuses on a clear intention for her work. She employs left brain critical-thinking skills while also attuning to right brain intuitions and artistic images.

An effective practitioner fosters her client's active participation in receiving the work. She encourages the client to pay attention to what is being done and to his own response to that work. The client is coached to invite the practitioner's hands into his sore, needy areas. Sometimes the client moves either in precisely guided patterns or in his own rhythm, thereby doing the work, in effect, for himself.

In the use of her own body, the practitioner must aim for yin/yang balance in order to be effective. The lower body—feet, legs, and pelvis—is best suited as the source of the yang qualities of strength, stability, balance, and endurance. Then the upper body—the torso, arms, hands, neck, and head—can relax fully into accessing the yin qualities of receptiveness to input, empathy, softness, and delicacy. Intention and focus can then be clearer.

Basic Principles Specific to Deep Tissue Sculpting

Attention to several principles specific to sculpting is necessary to effect the intended results of this method:

1. Pressure is usually applied parallel to muscle fibers, following the bone structure, or along fascial planes.
2. Compressions and strokes are performed with increasing pressure only to a level of balance between release and resistance.

3. Tissue change guides the speed, direction, and depth of all techniques.

Pressure is usually applied parallel to muscle fibers, following the bone structure, or along fascial planes

Since muscle fibers organize in a linear pattern, sculpting in the fiber direction naturally reorganizes the muscle. Areas that are disorganized into thickened tissue can be sculpted into line if pressure is applied parallel to the correctly aligned fibers. It is essential, then, for the practitioner to know precisely the origin, insertion, and direction of muscle fibers. This knowledge must be more than just intellectual; she must be able to visualize in her mind's eye a picture of the muscle being worked.

Often, the practitioner will be sculpting muscle in order to make contact with and bring consciousness to the bone structure

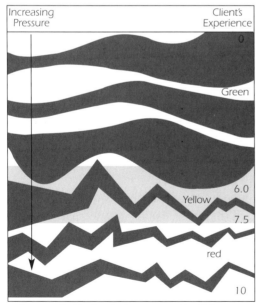

• **Image 6:** *Ideal sculpting pressure is mildly uncomfortable but predominantly pleasurable.*

beneath. Sometimes, release at the bony attachments of muscles is desired. When these are the intentions, then the practitioner must not only visualize the muscle, but also the bone beneath, and follow the bone as the structure that guides the sculpting tool.

Broad fascial sheaths and bands, such as the lumbodorsal fascia and the iliotibial tract, bind some body areas. They form intimately connected muscular and regional connective tissue units which Rolfer and anatomy instructor Tom Myers identifies as comprising seven lines of myofascial "trains."[5] These and the adjacent myofascial tissues become the focus of some fascial sculpting techniques.

Strokes and compression are done with increasing pressure only to a level of balance between release and resistance

The practitioner initiates a sculpting procedure by first applying light, then gradually increasing degrees of pressure to the chronically contracted tissue. Tissue yield and receptivity dictate the speed at which pressure is applied. Pressure is only applied to the level at which the client feels intensity, and not resistance, to the practitioner's touch. There may be pain involved, but it should have the flavor of pleasure on the borderline of pain, rather than pain with little pleasure. This level of experience is called the pleasure/pain line, the point of release, or the processing level of the tissue. In other words, change is occurring, but it is not so painful as to overwhelm the client in its intensity, nor is the touch so light that little or no change is accomplished. Too heavy sculpting pressure is destructive, and too light is ineffective and possibly boring to both client and practitioner. **(Image 6)**

Often, beginning practitioners like to use a feedback scale for developing their own sensitivity to this point of release. For example, she asks the client to report his perceived level of the sculpting intensity using numbers from 0 to 10. Zero indicates no sensation, intensity, or pain; five reflects a moderately intense sensation; 10 represents an overwhelming experience of pain, pressure, and intensity. Ideally the sculpting practitioner works at a perceived intensity level on this scale of 6.0 to 7.5. At that level of work, the client would be very aware of the tissue being touched and experience intense energy being introduced to the tissue. He might report some degree of pain, but it would have an "Oh, that hurts right" feel to it. He would feel the practitioner waiting for his tissue to relax.

Many clients work well with a color scheme for pleasure/pain verbal feedback that follows the common correlation of a traffic light. Green signifies completely pleasurable pressure, and red means more pain than pleasure. The most effective pressure level, where pleasure tinged with mild-discomfort-to-mild-pain is experienced, is coded as yellow.

Below this level, little lasting change will occur; above it, the client's body and psyche often feel violated and/or release is forced from the exterior rather than allowed from his interior. Forceful and abrupt movements also activate the client's defensive withdrawal reflexes that trigger increased muscular tension rather than relaxation. At high pain levels, the crossed extensor reflex activates the extensors of the opposite limb and may cause the entire body to push away from the source of pain. In determining appropriate pressure levels, it is helpful to remember that only in a receptive state can new behaviors, such as correct breathing, relaxation, and postural alignment be readily and thoroughly explored and learned.[6]

Tissue change guides the speed, direction, and depth of all techniques

Only energy being added to the tissue over time can elicit permanent relaxation of the myofascial tissues. This is due to the biomechanical properties of connective tissue discussed in the previous chapter. This necessarily means that deep tissue sculpting will proceed relatively slowly, compared to the most languid, Esalen-style circulatory massage. Some students' reactions to the slowness of this work led them to share a cartoon of a farmer preparing his field with a horse and plow. He comments, "Of course, I know what I'm doing—that's why it's taking me so long!"

When fascia and muscle release, there are a number of physical sensations that the sensitive practitioner can perceive:

- Hardness in the tissue may dissolve or melt, and the tissue feels softer
- The practitioner's tool may feel drawn deeper into the tissue as the fascia relaxes, much as the threads of a fabric spread with pressure
- An opening or spreading movement, or a pulsating or more fluid sensation

- A sensation of elongation of the muscles and a drawing of the practitioner's hand toward the elongation
- Heat generated by tissue release

All of these changes are palpable under the practitioner's hand, elbow, or forearm. Often it takes many hours of sculpting experience, the attentive and specific feedback of her client, and an exquisite openness to these subtle, often evasive sensations for a practitioner to confidently experience these tissue changes.

In addition, the observant practitioner can perceive other evidence of response:

- The client's breathing pattern may change, either increasing or decreasing in depth and speed.
- Either subtle or gross movements may begin stretching and manipulating the sculpted area from within, enhancing the reaction that the practitioner initiated.

- A visible elongation of the muscle or the entire body part being touched may occur.
- Jerking, twitching, and other omnidirectional movements may occur, either locally or in some distant area of the body as sculpting continues.
- Sometimes emotive reactions accompany the myofascial release in the form of sighing, crying, screaming, moaning, laughing, gesturing, or verbalization.

John Barnes, PT, developer of the Myofascial Release Seminars, adds his voice to other soft tissue practitioners in describing some of these phenomena as "unwinding." Barnes notes the tendency of the body to find a significant position, often the reproduction of or the opposite of the position in the moment of trauma that created the fascial constriction. A stillness often follows, and finally a release of myofascial restriction and feeling.[7]

Summary of Chapter Two

1. The practice of conscious bodywork is guided by four basic principles stating the assumptions, operating beliefs, and laws that determine its characteristics and outcomes.
2. By tuning in to the client with an intention to know, the practitioner is likely to choose the most appropriate techniques to meet the client's needs.
3. The more the practitioner is in the "ego-less" state of universal Love, the more able she is to receive all aspects of the client with empathy.
4. The clearer the practitioner's perception is of the client's needs and the clearer her intentions are for the work, then the more effective the work will be when the client is ready to receive it.
5. Natural, effortless movement between receptive and active energy within both the client and practitioner is the goal of many forms of body therapy.
6. Sculpting is most effective when guided by the basic principles governing the direction, depth, and speed of technique.
7. When applying pressure, the practitioner is guided by a clear image of the direction of the linear pattern of muscle fibers, of the bone to which the muscle is attached, and of the fascial planes involved.
8. To reach the point of release, the practitioner's pressure must be of sufficient intensity to register with the client but not be so intense as to cause the client to resist. This point is also known as the pleasure/pain line, the point of release, or the processing level of the tissue.
9. Since connective tissue releases relatively slowly with the gradual addition of pressure, the practitioner lets changes in the client's tissue and other observable responses in his body guide her work.

Sources Cited

[1] Maupin, Edward W., Ph.D. *The Structural Metaphor.* San Diego, CA: International Professional School of Bodywork, 2001.

[2] Maupin, Ibid, p.6.

[3] Galante, Laurence. *Tai Chi the Supreme Ultimate.* York Beach, ME: Samuel Weiser, Inc., 1981, p.28.

[4] Dychtwald, Ken. *Body-Mind.* New York, NY: Jove Publications, 1977, p.29.

[5] Myers, Thomas W. *Anatomy Trains: Myofascial Meridians for Manual and Movement Therapists.* Edinburgh, UK: Churchill Livingstone, 2001.

[6] Juhan, Deane. Job's Body: *A Handbook for Bodywork,* Expanded Edition. New York, NY: Station Hill Press, 1998, pp.208-209.

[7] Barnes, John F., P.T. "The Myofascial Release: Mind/Body Healing Approach," *Massage Magazine,* January/February, 1998, pp.91-94.

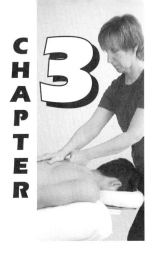

Structural Alignment and the Role of Injury and Illness in Back and Neck Pain

Balanced Structure:
To Heaven Above/Earth Below

The body is a sculpture formed around the framework of the bones. Skeletal elements provide a relatively solid base for creating a unique expression of curve, texture, proportion, density, and movement that is the individual human body. Yet, within so much individual variation, there are lines and planes characteristic of balanced, graceful, organized bodies.

The body's structure reveals the degree of balance of the soft tissues of the body: the muscles, fascia, tendons, and ligaments. Balanced structure reflects the body's efficiently organized response to the primary force of gravity. When efficiently organized, the body can use gravity as a source of uplifting and grounding energy rather than as an unrelenting drag.[1] Efficiently organized structure requires the muscles and fascia to be free of chronic tension, paired muscles to work in balanced opposition, muscles to function independently of their neighbors, and extrinsic and intrinsic muscles to be balanced in usage. But, how does one recognize balanced body structure?

A balanced body organizes around a central core of four gentle complementary spinal curvatures. The primary thoracic and sacral spinal curvatures are concave to the anterior, while the secondary cervical and lumbar curvatures are concave to the posterior. Although this is the commonly held view of the spine, there is debate among the various professionals who work with structure as to the optimum depth of these curvatures. For example, Ida Rolf recommended that vertebral elements be lined up one directly atop the other resulting in virtually no curvature.[2]

Among its various functions, the spine receives the weight of the upper body and distributes it to the pelvis and structures below. The vertebral elements must align so that the individual elements receive the weight evenly across the vertebral bodies. When there is excessive curvature, weight concentrates on the posterior or anterior portion of the various vertebrae. This uneven weight distribution produces excessive pressure on spinal nerves and on the intervertebral discs, and can result in disc damage. It also creates a variety of compensating misalignments throughout the head, and pectoral and pelvic girdles, as well as imbalance in the legs and feet.

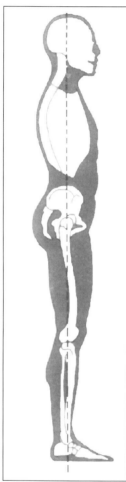

• **Image 7:** *balanced structural alignment on the vertical plane*

Shock absorption as the individual walks, runs, and moves about is another spinal function. When the spine is excessively curved, shock is unevenly distributed. A flattened curvature has diminished spring-like ability to absorb shock. Thus, gentle curvatures of all four areas of the spine are fundamental to balanced structure.

From a side perspective, practitioners can observe further evidence of balanced, integrated structure. An imaginary plumb line dropped through the crown of the aligned client's head shows alignment of the ear, the center of the shoulder, the greater trochanter of the femur, the lateral condyle of the knee, and the lateral ankle malleolus. **(Image 7)** If a plane is described down the posterior midline of the balanced body, a mid-sagittal plane, then all of the vertebral spinous processes will align along that plane. The nose and the navel also will align along the anterior midline. The balanced body reveals parallel, horizontal lines across the eyes, the clavicles, the iliac crests, and the knee and ankle joints. Finally, the anterior superior iliac spines and the symphysis pubis will align against a frontal plane. (See Maupin[3,] Myers[4,5] and Rolf[6] for further explanations of structural alignment principles.)

Many exercise methods, especially internally oriented methods such as yoga and tai chi chuan, encourage balanced spinal alignment. Tai chi practitioners imagine weight attaching to the coccyx. It pulls earthward and lengthens the spine, eliminating excess curvatures. A hook is simultaneously imagined as attaching to the crown of the head and continuing up toward the sky. This "skyhook" extends the spine, while it also aligns the head by tending to tuck the chin slightly. This complementary earthward and skyward extension of the spine creates lift and grounding in the individual's structure and energy field.

Common Structural Misalignments

Chronic muscle tension and the accompanying binding and pull on fascial planes produce much of the variety in human structure so evident in any observed group. While some individuals have straight, military-looking torsos, others are rounded and slumped. Many have upper or lower bodies that seem different from their other half, while some persons' left or right sides are elevated, rotated, or retracted from the midline, balanced position. Imbalance in paired and antagonist muscle groups and lack of independently functioning muscle neighbors also result in swaybacks, humpbacks, and other characteristic structural misalignments.

Flattened spinal curves

When the vertebral elements have little curvatures, then the curves appear flattened. Often the head retreats rigidly to the posterior on a straight cervical spine. Sometimes the chin juts forward as

Extremely tight erector spinae muscles bulging next to an anteriorly displaced, almost indiscernible, thoracic spine are the hallmark of a less common, but equally destructive, flattening of the thoracic curve.

Excessive spinal curves

An overly deep cervical or lumbar curvature is called lordosis. Cervical lordosis makes the neck appear shorter, and the head shift to the anterior on the atlas vertebrae. A lifted, anterior jutting chin usually accompanies this misalignment. **(Image 9)** With lumbar lordosis, or swayback, the pelvis also usually tilts so that the anterior superior iliac spines (ASIS) are anterior to the aligned frontal plane. **(Image 8 & 9)** Often both cervical and lumbar spine are lordotic.

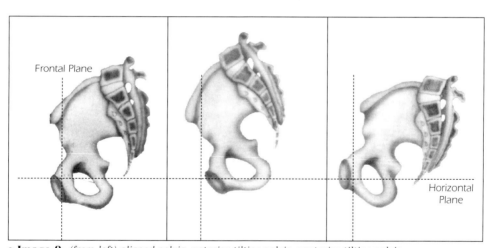

• **Image 8:** *(from left) aligned pelvis; anterior tilting pelvis; posterior tilting pelvis*

the cervical vertebrae are rigidly lined up, but pulled to the anterior as a whole spinal segment. Decreased lumbar curves also are common, accompanied usually by a posterior pelvic tilting evidenced by a flattened low back and buttocks. **(Image 8)**

Kyphosis describes the condition of excessive thoracic curvature. As the thoracic spine displaces to the posterior into this hunchbacked stance, the shoulders often round forward over a collapsed rib cage. **(Image 9)**

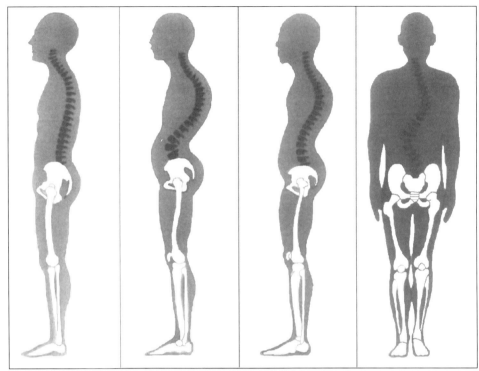

• **Image 9**: *(from left) cervical lordosis, lumbar lordosis, kyphosis, scoliosis*

Scoliosis

Soft tissue distortions can pull vertebral elements laterally from the midline of the body creating an S-shaped side curve called a scoliosis. Though sometimes congenital, scoliosis often develops during rapid adolescent growth. It can also result from degenerative disease or from excessive muscular tension, usually on the concave sides of the S-curve. Various pelvic and pectoral deviations usually occur in compensation for the scoliosis. **(Image 9)**

Misalignments of the head

In addition to the anterior and posterior imbalances of the occiput on the atlas described above, the head commonly misaligns into laterally tilted positions. The nose will not be on the body midline, and the horizontal line of the eyes and the chin will deviate. Rotation of the head toward a fixed left or right position also will appear to take the eyes and nose from a midline position. Careful observation should determine whether uneven eyes and other facial features are due to facial muscle tension or misalignment of the head and cervical spine. A complex combination of facial tension, rotations, tilting, and cervical misalignment is also common.

Pectoral and pelvic girdle misalignments

A pervasive imbalance in hectic urban societies is elevation of the pectoral girdle, with either unilateral or bilateral misalignment of the shoulders. The horizontal position of the clavicles gives way and results in the lateral end of the clavicles being higher than the sternal end. Viewed from the side, shoulders also either round and fall forward of the plumbline standard, or rigidly retract into a military posture of posterior displacement.

The shoulders and pelvis, as well as the head, are subject to rotational deviations and uneven tilts. Shoulder rotation, when one shoulder is forward of the plumbline standard and the other is posterior, is especially common with a scoliosis. One ASIS will be forward of the frontal plane, and the other ASIS will be posterior of that plane when the pelvis is rotated. Uneven iliac crest heights also are not unusual.

Evaluating Misaligned Structures

All of these misalignments are sometimes the result of misshapen bone, uneven lengths of the bones, or disease. More commonly, however, they reflect chronic muscle tension, connective tissue bunching, and/or imbalance in the functioning of paired muscles. The sculpting practitioner, therefore, must have a working knowledge of muscular and connective tissue structure, physiology, and kinesiology.[7] Then, with careful evaluation of a client's structure, he can determine the sites of most tension where sculpting proves most productive.

As an example, imagine that a client complains of tightness and discomfort in her left shoulder. Observation may reveal that her left shoulder appears elevated and rounded forward. To the knowledgeable practitioner, this can indicate that the left levator scapula, upper trapezius, pectoralis major, and pectoralis minor are chronically tensed. Another possibility, however, may be that the tense right latissimus dorsi, serratus anterior, lower trapezius, and erector spinae muscles, accompanied by glued posterior fascial sheaths, are dragging the right pectoral girdle inferior, so that the left side appears to be "higher." Successful results for this client will probably come from careful determination of which areas are causative of the misalignment, and then sculpting these specific structures.

Some of the many misalignments described above also are the result of imbalanced muscular function. Paired intrinsic/extrinsic muscles, such as the abdominals and psoas, and paired opposing muscles, such as the hamstrings group and the quadriceps group, often differ dramatically in their tone and/or tension levels. These types of imbalances are best addressed with sculpting techniques and perhaps stretches to release the chronically tightened muscle, and toning exercise for the underdeveloped, weaker muscle. For the example client above, toning the teres, rhomboids, latissimus, and lower trapezius also may help balance her elevated, anteriorly rotated left shoulder, thus freeing her of her discomfort.

Determining the causes of misalignment

"Even in my elementary school pictures I can see that I cocked my head over to this side and rolled my shoulders forward around my chest."

"My doctor says it's just arthritis, and it's to be expected by my age."

"I just bent over to pick up the newspaper, and suddenly I couldn't straighten up again."

"After a day's typing, the center of my back feels as though someone has a wrench in it and is constantly tightening it—and what a headache!"

"I've just never felt the same after that accident—constant headaches, tightness in my neck, and shoulders. Can you do anything for me?"

Each of these individuals presents typical complaints that lead U.S. consumers to over 114 million visits annually to massage therapists.[8] These practitioners regularly work with clients whose complaints range from generalized tension to extensive soft tissue involvement from injury or disease. While many clients describe very generalized complaints, the practitioner needs to be aware of the many possible causes that can lead to, "It just hurts right here."

Most people who seek deep tissue bodywork present complaints that are not pathological in origin. Chronic muscle spasm, acute muscle spasm, structural misalignment, overexertion, and mechanical low-back pain are the typical sources of clients' pain and complaints. Practitioners must always consider other, less common reasons for a client's discomforts. Injuries and illnesses will more often be involved for those practitioners who work with or on referral from doctors, osteopaths, chiropractors, and psychologists.

The practitioner's scope of practice in client evaluation

Ethical therapeutic massage and bodywork schools do not train students in diagnosis, nor are their graduates legally qualified to identify disease or injury. These functions are only within a physician's scope of practice. The bodywork practitioner may use the diagnosis of the client's medical doctor or osteopathic physician, or a chiropractor's evaluation to guide his work. If there is no diagnosis, and either he or his client has significant concern about possible injury or pathologies that may be involved, the practitioner should require a physician's examination before beginning body therapy.

Well-trained practitioners can evaluate their clients' posture and movement patterns. They have tuned and sharpened their eyes, hands, and kinesthetic senses to perceive nuances of restriction and imbalance in the musculoskeletal system. They often have received instruction in tests and examination procedures commonly used for diagnosis. (Consult Hoppenfield,[9] Benjamin,[10] and Travell and Simons[11] for detailed instruction in structural testing.) The bodywork practitioner, however, may only use these tests for guiding his own work, and not for diagnosing the client. This is, of course, often a difficult distinction for the practitioner to maintain, especially under pressure from the client to explain the reason for her pain.

The wise and ethical practitioner will:

- Take a complete physical and emotional history from his clients
- Inform clients of the contraindicated conditions for deep tissue work, and observe those contraindications
- Evaluate, within his own expertise, the possible causes for the client's complaint
- Refer, for a physician's diagnosis and possible treatment, those whose conditions indicate significant possibility of pathology
- Refrain from diagnosing clients' illnesses or injuries
- Communicate clearly with the client and her other healthcare providers the scope of his body therapy practice as legally and philosophically defined

The ideal: an integrative approach

Doctors, osteopaths, chiropractors, and physical therapists have been given the authority to treat disease and injury, some with limitations as to supervision and body areas. This is the usual emphasis of healthcare providers aligned to the rational philosophy of health care. It is the equally important, yet different, emphasis of empirical practitioners, such as therapeutic massage and bodywork practitioners, to nourish the body's vital energy. Hopefully, in the not-too-distant future, practitioners from both philosophies will integrate their approaches to client/patient care. Then, ideally the doctor will not only treat a patient's ruptured lumbar disc, for

example, but also will prescribe therapy that encourages the body's natural healing abilities. The massage and bodywork practitioner will not only relax chronic tension, thereby nourishing the body's energy, but also will refer for diagnosis and appropriate treatment, for example, the client whose straight leg raising test is positive for disc involvement.

An Outline of Causative Factors for Pain in the Back and Neck

The following limited outline is not intended for diagnostic purposes. It presents a detailed, though not exhaustive, list of the possible causes of pain in the back and neck. It includes a brief definition, implications for practitioners, types of bodywork and massage that typically work best with the condition, and any applicable contraindications or precautions. It includes only the back and neck since the primary emphasis of the hands-on work of this manual will be on these areas.

1. Chronic muscle spasm *Muscle in state of severe, involuntary contraction that extends over a period of time regardless of the need to accomplish a specific function.*
   a. can be the result of physical, emotional, or mental stress but is often emotional in origin, and then is known as "armoring"
   b. of a gradually increasing intensity and not usually of sudden onset
   c. often not felt as pain unless pressure is applied, but will be experienced as constant achiness, stiffness, or fatigue

d. responsive to heat and cold, and to deep tissue sculpting and other forms of bodywork

2. Acute muscle spasm *Muscle in state of severe, involuntary contraction that extends over a period of time, but is of sudden onset.*
   a. is extremely painful and often covers a broad muscular area
   b. occurs when tension overwhelms the muscle already in a state of chronic spasm, passing the body's tension limit; resulting pain inhibits further movement until recovery
   c. associated muscles also may be involved in a "splinting" capacity
   d. responds best to deep tissue and other neuromuscular types of bodywork, and to heat and cold

3. Structural/postural misalignments *Imbalances of the skeletal structure usually caused by chronic tension or incorrect movement habits.*
   a. responsive to deep tissue work and other bodywork
   b. some possible misalignments that produce back pain are tilting of the pelvis, lordosis, kyphosis, depressed chest, retracted shoulders, or elevated shoulders

4. Mechanical low-back pain *Chronic tension in the lumbar region due to uneven leg length, uneven pelvis, lumbar sacralization, structural scoliosis.*
   a. pain when the back is used, although rest will relieve the pain; pain is localized
   b. accompanied by muscle spasm in the low back, which is responsive to deep tissue sculpting and other bodywork

5. Overexertion *Pain resulting from physical activity, usually on a regular basis, such as that done by athletes, laborers, longshoremen, and childcare providers.*
   a. can produce other more serious back problems
   b. responsive to bodywork, especially deep circulatory massage, and to heat and cold

6. Somatic dysfunction *An impaired or altered function of related components of the somatic system (body framework), which includes the skeletal, arthroidial, and myofascial structures, and related vascular, lymphatic, and neural elements.*
   a. evaluation and diagnosis arrived at by observation of asymmetry of structures, decrease in range of motion, and quality of movement; also identified by palpable changes in tissue texture
   b. myofascial restriction and changes that accompany somatic dysfunction are particularly responsive to deep tissue sculpting and other forms of neuromuscular and myofascial techniques

7. Arthritis *Osteoarthritis involves wear and tear around the disc and facet joints of the vertebrae; spurs often build up along the joint.*
   a. results in mechanical low-back pain that tends to flare up periodically
   b. some accompanying muscle spasm that responds to bodywork, but avoid affected joints in acute stages
   c. rheumatoid arthritis and other forms of inflammatory joint disease such as ankylosing spondylitis and

gout can affect the muscular system with shortening of muscle fibers around affected joints; this often responds well to deep tissue sculpting, but should only be applied in nonacute stages

8. Muscle strain (tears and pulls)
   Stretching, tearing, or rupture of the muscle fiber.
   a. usually of sudden onset
   b. often accompanied by edema, and, when in the back, by paravertebral muscle spasm
   c. initially responds best to rest, ice, compression, and elevation (RICE), then to circulatory massage; after immediate edema and pain is reduced, responds to deep tissue sculpting and other forms of bodywork

9. Ligament sprain *Stretching, tearing, and rupture of ligament stretched beyond its strength.*
   a. more common in weight-bearing joints such as the ankle and knee, but also occurs in the back, particularly the cervical spine and pelvis
   b. accompanied by edema and associated tension in the surrounding musculature
   c. is not especially responsive to deep tissue sculpting, however, the associated muscle "splinting" is; RICE is effective
   d. cervical spine strain("whiplash"): occurs when the neck is driven into an extreme position, exerting tremendous pressure on the vertebral column and the

surrounding muscles and ligaments
   1) condition involves much "splinting" to hold the neck rigid so that the injured ligaments are not constantly aggravated
   2) often more on one side of the neck than the other
   3) often has a pain pattern of initial pain and then none after about 30 minutes; however, after several hours a dull aching begins that becomes very sharp and the entire neck spasms

10. Lumbar disc injuries ("slipped" disc, herniated or ruptured disc)
    Disintegration, dehydration, fragmentation, or abnormal pressure on the intervertebral discs, producing pressure on one or several nerves.
    a. most frequently involve the L-4 and L-5 discs
    b. accompanying pain from the buttocks traveling down the back of the leg indicates that the sciatic nerve is also being impinged; perhaps some numbness or pins-and-needles sensation as well
    c. associated muscle spasm around the injured disc, into the buttocks, and paravertebrally
    d. associated spasm responsive to deep tissue sculpting and other bodywork; use caution so that the injured disc will not be further pressured
    e. laminectomy, or removal of the bone fragments involved in a ruptured disc, is often performed

11. <u>Cervical spondylosis and cervical radiculitis</u> *Result of wear and tear in the spine, whereby the discs lose height and plumpness, allowing the vertebral bodies to move closer together, and leading to the formation of spurs around the injured area.*
    a. spurs pressure the cervical nerves, resulting in a pinched nerve or cervical radiculitis
    b. pain of gradually increasing intensity, which is constant and nagging, spreads along the shoulder to the top of the shoulder and the scapula, sometimes mimicking a heart attack by going into the chest area
    c. extreme stiffness in the neck responds to bodywork

12. <u>Acute cervical disc disease</u> *Fragmentation of the intervertebral disc, especially common between C-5 and C-6 and between C-6 and C-7.*
    a. pain will often spasm the neck muscles and radiate down one arm as the disc fragment impinges on a nerve
    b. associated spasm responds to bodywork; again use caution near the injured disc
    c. occasionally surgery, with subsequent immobilization of the neck with a collar, is performed and the resultant muscle spasm, adhesions, and decreased range of motion (ROM) respond to bodywork

13. <u>Spondylolysis and Spondylolisthesis</u> *A loosened vertebra and slipping of a vertebral element.*
    a. usually involves the L-5 vertebral element
    b. spondylolysis starts as a crack in the arch portion of the vertebra; when the arch cracks through, it is then free to slide forward on the element just below it, causing spondylolisthesis
    c. usually accompanied by an insidiously increasing low back pain going straight across the back itself that seldom radiates into the legs
    d. very tight hamstring group and associated spasms in the erector spinae, which respond to deep tissue sculpting and other forms of bodywork
    e. degree of spondylolisthesis is important to know so that no bodywork that presses against the slipped portion is applied
    f. often treated surgically with a spinal fusion; spasm, muscle shortening, adhesions, and decrease in ROM following surgery are responsive to bodywork

14. <u>Fracture</u> *Breaking of a bone.*
    a. almost always of sudden onset
    b. accompanied by edema and associated muscle tension/splinting
    c. recovery involves restoring ROM and lengthening of muscle and ligaments
    d. bodywork in the area is contraindicated until after the fracture has healed; in cervical and other spinal fractures, proceed only

with extreme caution and after consultation with the physician

e. associated muscle tension is responsive to deep tissue sculpting, and edema is responsive to circulatory massage

15. Tumor and infection
    a. although few cases of back and neck pain presented to the bodywork practitioner will be the result of tumors pressing on the spinal nerves or embedded in the musculature, this possibility should be considered; deep tissue sculpting is generally contraindicated; thorough consultation with medical professionals and careful decision-making regarding other forms of massage therapy (nothing except the very lightest, soothing touch) is critical
    b. bacterial and viral infections, such as osteomyelitis, can affect the muscle, connective tissue, bone and/or joints of the body

16. Other diseases, disorders, abnormalities and congenital deformities
    a. in some disorders, circulating antibodies or cell-mediated immunity can result in muscle fiber injury or destruction, or adhesion formation such as in polymyositis; sensitive deep tissue sculpting and cross-fiber deep tissue techniques are effective, carefully monitoring client response
    b. other joint abnormalities such as gout, infectious arthritis, and repeated hemorrhage, as in

hemophilia, can cause pain

c. congenital abnormalities and developmental injuries, disorders, and defects such as muscular torticollis, dislocated hips, cerebral palsy, and clubfoot can result in back and neck pain; resulting shortened soft tissue and tension generally respond well to sculpting

d. metabolic bone diseases, such as osteoporosis, produce changes in the bony structure; resultant chronic muscle tension responds well to sculpting, but caution should be taken with deep pressures due to bone fragility

e. diseases of the muscle motor unit include muscular dystrophies, neuropathies, and spinal muscular atrophies such as poliomyelitis; these diseases can cause pain due to muscular atrophy and decreased ROM; they respond best to circulatory and passive joint methods of bodywork, but also to careful deep tissue sculpting

17. Myofascial syndromes
    a. aching tender muscles with tender points that often refer pain to other sites are called trigger points; studied most extensively by Janet Travell, M.D., these points are quite likely many of the painful areas encountered while sculpting; while medical treatment of trigger points usually involves injections of cortisone and local anesthetics, deep tissue sculpting is particularly effective in erasing these points, as are the specific techniques of

manual erasure of these points accompanied by stretching

b. generalized achiness, muscle spasm, and tiredness accompanied by hard nodular localized areas and predictable tender points characterize fibromyalgia (fibrositis or myodysneuria). Deep tissue sculpting is often too intense, but sensitive, gentle, limited applications of sculpting can be effective; proceed conservatively and with detailed client feedback[12]

Summary of Chapter Three

1. A balanced body structure responds efficiently to gravity. Its spine extends both earthward and skyward along four gentle complementary curves and its soft tissue is free from chronic tension.

2. Much of the variation seen in human structures is due to structural misalignments that happen when chronic muscle tension and shortened fascial planes pull on the bones.

3. When the vertebral elements have no gentle curvatures, that part of the spine is flattened.

4. An excessive cervical or lumbar curvature, for example a swayback, is called lordosis. Excessive thoracic curvature is called kyphosis.

5. Scoliosis is characterized by an S-shaped side curve of the spine, and occurs when the vertebral elements are pulled laterally from the midline of the body, often during rapid adolescent growth.

6. The head often presents complex combinations of rotations, tiltings, and other cervical misalignments in addition to the anterior/posterior imbalance of the occiput on the atlas.

7. In the pectoral girdle, misalignments which are often caused by stress include raised and rounded shoulders and a constricted rib cage. Both the shoulders and the pelvis are also subject to rotational deviations and uneven tilts.

8. The practitioner must use his knowledge of muscular and connective tissue and kinesiology to evaluate misalignments in his client's structure and determine the sites of tension that will benefit most from sculpting.

9. While most clients' complaints are not pathological, the practitioner still needs to be aware of the many possible causes of pain and tension, particularly if he is working with clients who have been ill or injured.

10. Although the practitioner's training and scope of practice do not allow him to diagnose disease or injury, he must still carry out a thorough evaluation of the client, including referral to a physician when necessary.

11. In an ideal, integrative approach to health care, practitioners from both the rational and empirical models would each play roles in both treating the presenting problem and nourishing the body's vital healing energy.

Sources Cited

[1] Rolf, Ida P., Ph.D. Rolfing: *The Integration of Human Structures*. New York, NY: Harper and Row, 1977, pp.29-34.

[2] Feitis, Rosemary, Editor. *Ida Rolf Talks About Rolfing and Physical Reality*. New York, NY: Harper and Row, 1978, p.74.

[3] Maupin, Edward W., Ph.D. *The Structural Metaphor: An Introduction to the Rolf Method of Structural Integration* (Part One and Two). San Diego, CA: International Professional School of Bodywork, 2001.

[4] Myers, Thomas W. "Body Cubed" (article series). *Massage Magazine* Issues September/October, 1997-January/February, 2000.

[5] Myers, Thomas W. *The Anatomy Trains: Myofascial Meridians for Manual and Movement Therapists*. Edinburgh, UK: Churchill Livingstone, 2001

[6] Rolf, Op. Cit.

[7] For an excellent reference book illustrating anatomy and its functional relationship to actual movements in daily activities, dance and exercise, see: Calais-Germain, Blandine. *Anatomy of Movement*. Seattle, WA: Eastland Press. 1993.

[8] Eisenberg, et. al. "Trends in Alternative Medicine Use in the United States, 1990-1997." *Journal of the American Medical Association* 280(18): November 11, 1998, pp.1569-1575.

[9] Hoppenfeld, Stanley. *Physical Examination of the Spine and Extremities*. New York, NY: Appleton-Century-Crofts, 1976.

[10] Benjamin, Ben, Ph.D. with Gale Borden, M.D. *Listen to your Pain*. New York, NY: Penguin Books, 1987.

[11] Travell, Janet G., M.D. and David G. Simons, M.D. *Myofascial Pain and Dysfunction*, Volumes One and Two. Baltimore, MD: Williams and Wilkins, 1992.

[12] Sources for this outline include:
   Benjamin, Ben E., Ph.D. *Are You Tense?* New York, NY: Pantheon Books, 1978. Chapters 1 and 7, and Lessons One-Five.

   Cailliet, Rene, M.D. *Soft Tissue Pain and Disability*. Philadelphia, PA: F.A. Davis Co., 1977. Chapters 1-4.

   Chaitow, Leon, N.D., D.O. *Modern Neuromuscular Techniques*. Edinburgh, Scotland: Churchill Livingstone, 1996.

   Curties, Debra. *Massage Therapy and Cancer*. New Brunswick, Canada: Curties-Overzet Publications, Inc., 1999.

   Hoppenfield, Stanley, M.D. *Physical Examination of the Spine and Extremities*. New York, NY: Appleton-Century Crofts, 1976. Chapters 4, 6, 9.

   Rosse, Cornelius, M.D., and D. Kay Clawson, M.D. *The Musculoskeletal System in Health and Disease*. New York, NY: Harper and Row, 1980, Chapter 6, pp.20-29.

   Southmayd, William, M.D., and Marshall Hoffman. *Sportshealth: The Complete Book of Athletic Injuries*. New York, NY: Quick Fox, 1981, Chapters 3-5, 10, and 11.

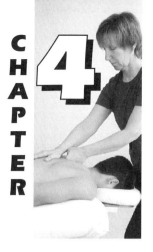

CHAPTER 4

Body/Mind: The Role of Emotions in Chronic Tension and Pain

Historical and Research Perspectives

For thousands of years ancient traditions have explored the connections between the body, the emotions, and the intellect. Religions, health practices, and many cultural and educational institutions of China, India, and other Eastern countries reflect a holistic perspective, a sense of the interconnectedness between the body and the mind, and, indeed, between the individual and the entire macrocosm. Many of the earliest Western cultures, including the earth-based traditions of the Celts and indigenous American cultures, also embraced similar paradigms.[1, 2] Mainstream Western tradition, dominated by Christianity for nearly two thousand years, has, on the other hand, upheld separation of the mind and the body as the dominant model of humanity. Dualism, as propounded by French philosopher Descartes in the 1600s, has characterized modern Western thinking and healthcare.

On the other hand, body-oriented psychotherapy has evolved over the last

century to a viable perspective in promoting the health of the entire individual. Wilhelm Reich and Carl Jung in the late 1920s pioneered these explorations. Reconnection with and investigation of the body/mind concept began in earnest in the West during the 1960s. Fritz Perls formulated Gestalt therapy, and in the '60s and '70s Reich's students, Alexander Lowen, John Pierrakos, and William Walling, developed Reich's work into the recognized psychological techniques of bioenergetics. Psychologists, physicians, researchers, and most "human potential movement" participants began acknowledging the shared consciousness of the mind and body.

Psychology with a somatic perspective, the integral interaction between the physical body, the emotions, and the soul, has become a growing and vital paradigm in contemporary psychotherapy. Although the use of touch in psychoanalysis is embroiled in discussions of its impact on transference-countertransference dynamics and sexual ethics, some therapists and other mental health practitioners integrate the two. Among the most widely known are Arthur Janov, Ilana Rubenfeld, and Marion Woodman.[3] Peter Levine[4] and Ron Kurtz[5] also recently have made vibrant contributions to this subsection of psychological treatment. Other therapists have articulated a psychophysical model with a collaborative team of a psychotherapist and a bodyworker at its foundation.[6,7]

Doctors have also begun to express a deeper appreciation for the mind's subtle, yet systemic effects on physical health. *New York Times* #1 bestseller, *Spontaneous Healing*, written by Andrew Weil, a Harvard trained physician, advocates using the intricate interaction of the mind and body, as well as medical treatment and other lifestyle changes, to resolve life-threatening diseases, severe trauma, and chronic pain.[8] Fritz Frederick Smith, M.D., Leon Chaitow D.O., and John Upledger, D.O. are all internationally known physicians/authors whose treatment methodologies and protocols deeply acknowledge the fundamental connections of the feeling body and the physical body. In addition, chiropractor Clyde Ford[9] and physical therapist John Barnes[10] are noteworthy examples of other healthcare providers whose theoretical frameworks are holistically or somatically oriented.

A recent explosion of reputable scientific research suggests that the mind and body act on each other in remarkable ways. Scientific research into the connection between the brain and the immune system, a new discipline called psychoneuroimmunology, or PNI, flourishes at the University of Michigan, the University of Pennsylvania, Ohio State University College of Medicine, and the National Institute of Mental Health, as well as other respected institutions.[11]

Candace Pert is one of this growing number of medical researchers and practitioners whose work is reshaping the perspective of traditional Western medicine. Her discoveries recognize the interconnectedness of Western medicine's various branches, e.g., neurology, virology, immunology, psychology. Her research results demonstrate beyond any doubt that the human being is itself an interconnected holistic entity. Through her work with neuropeptides, receptors, ligands, and other "informational substances," Pert establishes conclusively that there is such a thing as the bodymind and that it exists at the molecular level. The intricate process carried on by these informational substances operates across all body systems, and includes emotions, memories, bodily sensations, and habitual patterns, and plays a key role in health and healing. Of importance for deep tissue practitioners, Pert asserts in her book, *Molecules of Emotion*, that "usually this process takes place at an unconscious level, but it can also surface into consciousness under certain conditions, or be brought into consciousness by intention."[12] This is certainly the reality which bodyworkers, massage therapists, and other touch specialists feel beneath their hands: chronically constricted muscles often reflect chronically constricted emotions.

The late Thomas Hanna, Ph.D., coined the term *somatics* (from the Greek, soma, or living body) and was one of the earliest authors to articulate a somatic wellness perspective.[13] Somatics was developed by Hanna's Novato Institute for Somatic Research and Training. Various other body therapy schools call this perspective somatic integration. By either name, it views a human as not only the physical body subject to physical and organic forces, but also as the inner, experiencing being who can change himself.[14] The somatic concept of the feeling body in careful self-observation has parallels in the therapies and dance and movement educational systems of Rudolph Von Laban, Moshe Feldenkrais, Mary Starks Whitehouse, Gerda and F.M. Alexander, and Judith Aston.[15]

Although most known for her insights and techniques of structural integration, Ida Rolf recognized that integration of structure moves the client to experience "the basic link that exists between structure and emotion."[16] Many of Rolf's students, including Ed Maupin, Tom Myers, Joseph Heller, Michael Shea, and Fritz Fredrick Smith, have elaborated on and developed the concepts of structural bodywork to affect the mind. The proliferation in recent years of articles and entire journals exploring somatic themes in therapeutic massage and bodywork attests to the intense interest and recognition of this sensibility in the touch professions.

Storing Emotions in the Body

Many bodywork practitioners note that even the most physical complaint presented by a client usually has a conscious or unconscious emotional component. Rare, indeed, is the individual who can, for example, sustain a cervical strain injury without some degree of fear, sadness, or anger associated with the precipitating event. When relief from the physical trauma of injury or illness is sought, release of associated emotions is often necessary for full recovery.

For example, as the brakes are slammed on, and the car is skidding, Catie's last thoughts before impact with the stalled car before her are, "Oh, my God, I'm going to die!" She gasps, holding her breath, awaiting the inevitable. A return to consciousness finds her with a broken leg and head injuries, but she is alive. Shock, pain, and attention to her physical needs distract her from a vague awareness of an underlying fear and her shallow breathing. The next day, casted and stitched, she returns home. The safety of home and family may immediately loosen fearful tears. Between sobs and wails, she might recount the details of the accident until her breath deepens, her fear is spent, and only then does she feel relieved. On the other hand, the trauma of this threat may stay with her for many decades.

Emotional trauma sustained in accidents, loss of loved ones, violent natural or interpersonal experiences, and repeated abuse or deprivation often profoundly impact the body's soft tissue. Even a moderately sensitive person can observe any group of people and identify anger, sadness, or fear in habitually stooped postures or chest-inflated poses. Psychologists and psychiatrists treat emotionally disturbed patients, whose bodies are often twisted and frozen into graphic expressions of the solidified feelings that torment these individuals.

Peter Levine's *Waking the Tiger* details humans' similarity to reptiles and other mammals in their response to an overwhelming threat: fight, flight, or freeze. The freeze response, or physical immobility, is similar to the "playing possum" of a captured animal as its predator controls it. Levine contends that this frozen energy, if left unresolved and not discharged, remains in the nervous system creating residual traumatic symptoms including anxiety, depression, and many psychosomatic and behavioral problems.[17]

In addition to accidents and violent experiences, a typical mother-child interaction exemplifies how developmental events can affect structure and physiology. Two-year-old Timothy curiously explores his mother's jewelry, delighting in the feel of the cool metals, the sparkle of the rhinestones. Upon discovery, Mom sternly says, "No!," slaps Timothy's hands, and angrily secures her treasures. Timothy responds to Mom's anger and restriction with startled breath holding, retracting his hands, and ducking his head in fear. Shallow breathing continues as Mom rages. Later, as things quiet down, Timothy's breathing becomes more normalized, and his pudgy hands reach out again in relentless investigation of the world.

If this and other angry, fearful interactions occur regularly, however, Timothy may become constantly fearful and apprehensive of his mother's restriction and anger. Chronically shallow breathing may reflect tension in the diaphragm and chest. Pectoralis, teres, rhomboids, and latissimus may retain a level of contraction in an attempt to hold his hands back from the impulsive exploration that provokes the feared anger from his mother. His chest may become collapsed and his shoulders rounded in an expression of crushed love and fearful self-protection. Chronic emotional stress becomes chronic muscular stress.

The Bodywork Practitioner's Role in Somato-emotional Integration

Respectful, loving awareness of feelings and acceptance of them is the essential nature of human beings and a hallmark of an effective bodywork practitioner. Maintaining an accepting, respectful relationship with a client often creates a context that evokes emotional expression. This expression is not necessarily dramatic and graphic. A heartfelt but single sigh, a brief outburst of feeling, or a silent, solitary tear can communicate profoundly.

The body awareness generated by deep sculpting and other conscious body therapies can short-circuit the usual physical and intellectual defenses, and emotions can emerge from hiding. Clients sometimes experience waves of strong sadness or vague whispers of long-ago

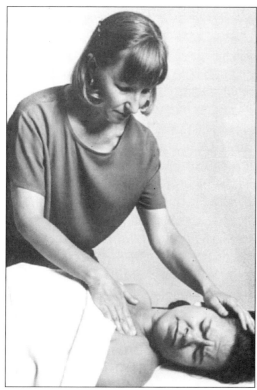

• **Image 10**: *The practitioner emotionally supports her client by guiding the client's breath and focusing her own awareness.*

fears as sensitive hands touch them. Sometimes clients tense up even more to defend from long-suppressed feelings surfacing during their sessions. Awareness and acceptance of these emotional responses usually facilitates the relaxation of tension in the myofascial tissues. It also promotes an integration of the client's physical, emotional, and intellectual experience of his being.

The practitioner who uses deep tissue sculpting must be more alert and comfortable with emotional responses than when using some other systems of body therapy. The intensity of physical sensation, as chronic tension is met with

focused pressure, often provokes corresponding emotional intensity. Deep sighs, moans, grunts, tears, screaming, striking, kicking, or flailing to express these feelings are all possibilities. The bodywork practitioner need not "do" anything with or about her clients' emotions, unexpressed or expressed, other than be a loving human being. **(Image 10)** As a supplement to respectful love, a few techniques for increasing or decreasing emotional expression often are useful to the sculpting practitioner.

Encouraging Expression

Tears or sounds may surface on their own. However, due to strong societal training in the repression of negativity, some clients need explicit permission to resolve their tensions in this way. Expression can be facilitated by verbal encouragement: "Can you let your tears come?" "Can you let it be okay for you to feel this?" Touch, such as stroking a trembling chin or gently rubbing the belly, provides tactile communication that these feelings are acceptable. Increasing the pressure of sculpting techniques so that slightly more pain is experienced can sometimes loosen feelings that are about to emerge but need more propulsion to fully appear.

The breath is the link between the body and the emotions. Reich's observations led him to think that "the inhibition of respiration is the physiological mechanism of suppression and repression of emotion, and was thus the basic mechanism of neurosis in general. The diaphragmatic contraction is an early physical move to suppress sensation, whether of pleasure or anxiety… [and] had the biological function of reducing the production of energy in the organism, which supposedly leads to a lessening of anxiety."[18]

The sensitive bodywork practitioner utilizes this knowledge with her clients. Changes in the client's breathing pattern should always alert the practitioner to a change in response to work. When the breath deepens, the client may be just falling asleep. Sleep is sometimes a protective response to intense feelings; however, deeper and/or more rapid breathing usually heralds surfacing emotions. Holding the breath or breathing shallowly sometimes occurs instead.

To facilitate the release of emotions when there is a breath change that signals emotional response, sustained pressure at the solar plexus is very effective. Requesting that exhales be through slightly parted lips also opens expression through the mouth. The verbal instruction, "Breathe," can encourage both breathing and emotional expression. Signs of tetany and/or hyperventilation, when breathing is rapid or inhales deeper than exhales, need to be monitored by observing the client's hands and mouth. These signs include: numbness, stiffness, or tingling around the mouth and in the distal parts of any extremity; dizziness; lightheadedness; and visual disturbances. If necessary, the practitioner's cupped hands, a paper bag, or a cup placed over the client's mouth can help to resolve the oxygen-carbon dioxide imbalance that occurs if the client continues to hyperventilate.

Decelerating Expression

While acceptance of emotions is a necessity, expression may not always be appropriate or safe. Some clients will not seem stable enough to healthily integrate intense feelings. Practitioners should carefully interview and evaluate clients regarding their emotional and physical health. When working with clients with a history of prior psychotherapeutic or psychiatric care, and those currently in therapy, consultation with the psychotherapist or physician usually should be sought. This is especially important when working with someone who is also in the detoxification stages of substance abuse, or anytime there are indications of psychological instability. Some clients will not feel comfortable or confident with emotional expression. Physical limitations, such as pain, casting, or injuries that may be aggravated by forceful movement, may preclude any kicking or hitting of cushions or table with angry releases.

Lack of confidence, training, or skill may limit the practitioner's willingness to work with emotional expression. Limitations in noise level, stability of therapy table, or other environmental restraints may need to be respected. Lack of time to achieve closure with an emotional process also should lead the practitioner to limit emotional expression. A physically small practitioner working with a large client often feels that only sounds, words, tears, and other less physical expressions are manageable to protect both herself and the client. It is usually safest to work at an emotional level with clients who have a viable support network of family, friends, groups, and/or professionals.

If the practitioner feels any restrictions to the free expression of feelings, these should be clearly and sensitively communicated to the client when emotional response is first perceived. The practitioner can then assist her client in backing off from emotive response with several effective techniques. Engaging the client's intellect usually successfully stifles emotional movement. Exploration of the issues generated can perhaps continue by talking of them in more intellectual terms. The practitioner may ask, "Why do you feel sad?", rather than the more provocative, "Your sadness seems very deep." If more complete shutdown of the emotions seems necessary, then discussing nonpersonal topics is usually effective. Requesting that the client open his eyes, reorient to the current environment, or breathe more deeply into the abdomen also can effectively tone down emotional response.

Decreasing the pressure and intensity of the sculpting, or using another, more superficial technique, also can decrease emotional intensity. Sometimes the area that retains the emotional charge needs to be left, and the session must proceed to other body parts. Firm, but gentle, holding of the feet is usually effective for reducing emotional response. In some cases, the practitioner will have to stop the session completely in order to respect her own or her client's limits on emotional expression.

Emotional release in conjunction with deep tissue sculpting or any other bodywork modality should be viewed as a possibility, but neither inevitable nor required. Client and practitioner must proceed with emotional expression only with mutual consent and respect. Attention to limitations in the practitioner's scope of practice and in her expertise is crucial, and the treatment of mental illness may only be pursued by those professionally trained and licensed to do so.

Psychological Correspondences and Body/Mind "Maps"

Sensitivity to the language of the body is a critical skill for the conscious bodywork practitioner to develop. Visual, audible, tactile, and kinesthetic clues in the client's structure, words, and movement can reveal feelings, beliefs, and thought patterns that reflect the unique individual beneath her hands. This knowledge can be useful when sculpting to release chronic myofascial tension.

Observation and clinical experience have led some psychologists and other practitioners to devise representations, or body/mind maps, of expected or common correlations between the body's language and feelings. Reich's theoretical descendents Kurtz and Prestera,[19] Dychtwald,[20] and Keleman[21] each articulated theories of structural functions/dysfunctions and physical and emotional holding patterns correlated to individual body and psychological types. If utilizing such maps of correspondences between physical and emotional tensions, the practitioner must remember that the truth of what an individual's body reflects is found in that person, not within a theory. Internal and verbal questioning of imbalanced areas should be done using body/mind theories as clues and probabilities, not verities.

Theories concerning the body areas taught in this manual are included with each session chapter. Various body/mind maps are detailed by other authors, such as those noted above. Training programs and instructors at some therapeutic massage and bodywork schools also use these types of maps. Others, notably the International Professional School of Bodywork, Canadian Matthew van der Giessen's Somatic Arts Institute, and Ron Kurtz's Hakomi Institute offer practitioners a more open-ended, experiential paradigm of somatic psychology. The psychological perspective initially taught in the 1970s by the Arica Institute is equally brilliant, but less widely known.

Arica Institute Perspective on Body Psychology

An eclectic school of knowledge of transformative traditions and technologies, the Arica Institute formed in 1968 in response to the experience of 52 individuals with a Bolivian mystic and teacher, Oscar Ichazo. Gathered in Arica, Chile, where Ichazo was living, they entreated him to teach them the various esoteric and consciousness-altering techniques that he had been studying since his early teens with masters of martial arts, shamanism, philosophy, Zen, Sufism, Kaballah, and Gurdjieff.

Ichazo's teachings and the contributions of the many psychologists, artists, and other professionals in that first training, and in subsequent ones, has evolved into a nine-tiered system of trainings and practices. The school has contemporized the ancient methods of enlightenment with the insights of biology, psychology, and physics to create a comprehensive method designed to clarify the human process into states of enlightenment and true liberation. Arica™ trainings are currently offered in locations around the world, and the Institute headquarters in Connecticut disseminates information and materials and offers trainings, many by mail order.[22]

Arica presents powerful theories and maps to increase understanding of the human body and psyche. Of particular usefulness to the psychologically sensitive bodyworker are those correlating physical and emotional/psychological functions. These include: the ego fixations and enneagons[sm], the Nine Hypergnostic Systems[sm], the Levels of Consciousness[sm], the Domains of Consciousness[sm], and the Chua K'a[sm] correspondences of body/emotional fears.

Oscar Ichazo explained his perspective on the formation of ego and personality in a 1973 interview first published in *Psychology Today:*

> In essence, every person is perfect, fearless, and in a loving unity with the entire cosmos; there is no conflict within their person between head, heart, and stomach or between the person and others. Every human being starts in pure essence. Then something happens: the ego begins to

develop; karma accumulates; there is a transition from objectivity to subjectivity; man falls from essence into personality....a contradiction develops between the inner feelings of the child and the outer social reality to which he must conform....When we turn away from our primal perfection, our completeness, our unity with the world and God, we create the illusion that we need something exterior to ourselves for our completion. This dependency on what is exterior is what makes man's ego.[23]

Becoming Psychologically Sensitive

Explanation or reading alone, of course, cannot bring about knowledge and embodiment of somatic theories. Participation in integrative somatic-oriented programs, such as those mentioned in this chapter, or in personal somatic therapy, is recommended. After incorporating studied techniques into her life, the bodywork practitioner can expect to more accurately understand and identify body/mind correspondences. Once internalized, they are of vast usefulness to the psychologically sensitive practitioner.

Summary of Chapter Four:

1. The ancient teachings of the East have traditionally explored the interconnection of mind/body/emotions. More recently, notable Western researchers and practitioners, particularly those in the field of psychotherapy and within the "human potential" and holistic health movements, also have embraced this interconnection.

2. Even the most physical complaint presented by a client usually has an emotional component, be it conscious or unconscious.

3. The psychologically sensitive practitioner is prepared for the possibility of the client's release of emotions and provides skillful and respectful support to help the client integrate his experiences.

4. The practitioner can help the client retrieve and safely express his feelings through her verbal encouragement, tactile communication and pressure, and by keeping the client focused on his breath.

5. During a sculpting session, a client may need to back off from free expression of his feelings due to limitations such as the practitioner's skill level, the client's own condition, the physical setting, or time constraints. The practitioner helps him do this through appropriate verbal and touch contact.

6. Knowing the language of the body and its correspondences with psychological patterns can be useful for the practitioner who is releasing a client's chronic myofascial tension.

7. The Arica Institute is an eclectic school of transformative traditions and technologies which presents powerful theories and maps for understanding the human body and psyche, pure human essence, ego formation and correspondences of body/emotional fears.

Sources Cited

[1] Smolen, Rick, Phillip Moffitt, and Matthew Naythons, M.D. *The Power to Heal: Ancient Arts and Modern Medicine.* New York, NY: Prentice Hall Press, 1990.

[2] Guinness, Alma E., editor. *Family Guide to Natural Medicine.* Pleasantwille, NY: Reader's Digest Association, Inc., 1993.

[3] van der Giessen, Matthew J. "Psyche and Soma," *Massage Therapy Journal.* Summer, 1990, pp. 67-72.

[4] Levine, Peter, Ph. D. with Ann Frederick. *Waking the Tiger: Healing Trauma.* Berkeley, CA: North Atlantic Books, 1997.

[5] Kurtz, Ron. *Body-Centered Psychotherapy: The Hakomi Method.* Mendocino, CA: LifeRhythm, 1990.

[6] Timms, Robert, Ph.D., and Patrick Connors, CMT. *Embodying Healing: Integrating Bodywork and Psychotherapy in Recovery from Childhood Sexual Abuse.* Orwell, VT: Safer Society Press, 1992.

[7] Mower, Melissa B. "The Team Approach to a Body/Mind Session." *Massage Magazine*: Jan-Feb., 1998, Issue 71, pp.32-39.

[8] Weil, Andrew, M.D. *Spontaneous Healing.* New York, NY: Ballantine Books, 1995.

[9] Ford, Clyde. *Compassionate Touch.* Park Ridge, IL: Parkside Publishing, 1993.

[10] Barnes, John F. *Healing Ancient Wounds: The Renegade's Wisdom.* Paoli, PA : Rehabilitation Services, Inc., 2000.

[11] "Body and Soul." *Newsweek*: November 7, 1988, pp.88-90.

[12] Pert, Candace B., Ph.D. *Molecules of Emotion.* New York, NY: Scribner, 1997, p.142.

[13] Hanna, Thomas, Ph.D. *Somatics.* Reading, MA: Addison-Wesley Publishing Co. Inc., p.21.

[14] For integrative somatics educational programs contact: International Professional School of Bodywork, 1366 Hornblend St. San Diego, CA 92109, 858-272-4142. www.IPSB.com. Also contact: Hakomi Institute, PO Box 1873, Boulder, CO 80306.

[15] McNeely, Deldon Anne, Ph.D. *Touching: Body Therapy and Depth Psychology.* Toronto, Canada: Inner City Books, 1987, pp.27-51.

[16] Rolf, Ida, Ph.D. *Rolfing.* Rolf Institute: Boulder, CO, 1977, p.17.

[17] Levine, Op. Cit., pp.15-21.

[18] Reich, Wilhelm. *The Function of the Orgasm.* New York, NY: World Publishing, 1942, p.267.

[19] Kurtz, Ron, and Hector Prestera. *The Body Reveals.* New York, NY: Harper and Row, 1976.

[20] Dychtwald, Ken. *Bodymind.* Los Angeles, CA: Tarcher, 1986.

[21] Keleman, Stanley. *Emotional Anatomy.* Berkeley, CA: Center Press, 1985.

[22] For information on the Arica Institute programs, contact: Arica Institute, Inc., 10 Landmark Lane, Kent, Connecticut, 06757. orders@arica.org

[23] Keen, Sam. "We have no desire to strengthen the ego or make it happy," an interview with Oscar Ichazo. *Psychology Today*, July, 1973.

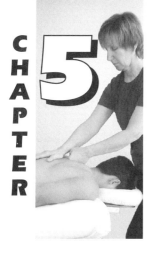

CHAPTER 5

How to Sculpt

The first two chapters of this manual explained what sculpting is and explored how it works. Chapter Three explored the basics of structural integrity, describing how structural misalignments, injuries and illnesses contribute to neck and back pain. Somatic integration, the inner awareness of the connection between feelings, thoughts, and experiences and bodily sensation, were the focus of Chapter Four. With an understanding of these concepts you now are ready to learn to apply them and to learn how to sculpt.

Practitioner's Skill Development

To practice deep tissue sculpting effectively, you must develop skills in the following areas:
- Understanding the client: learning to observe, to analyze, and to listen and intuit holistically so that clear session intentions evolve
- Body mechanics: using your body economically and appropriately
- Technique: sensitively entering and exiting your client's body, choosing appropriate "tools," and controlling your work

- Receptivity and responsiveness: responding to your client's level of release, connecting empathetically and intuitively, and focusing on intention

These next two chapters will guide you in developing these skills.

Understanding your Client

Before ever touching your client's body, you must first "read" areas of tension and evaluate your client. This involves four very important steps: observing and perceiving; analyzing; intuiting; and finally, clarifying and visualizing overall session and procedural intentions.

Observing and perceiving the client

The client reveals to the observant practitioner many clues to her needs. These clues can guide you to appropriate work. Visual observation yields information about:
- Postural balance and imbalance
- Movement patterns
- Contracted, shortened soft tissue
- Expressions of emotional tension
- Signs of muscle imbalance or deterioration

• Clues to pain patterns

Customary client profiles or intake questionnaires that include health history, current complaints, and desired session outcomes offer a wealth of concrete information. When you discuss this data with your client and hear her concerns, you can learn much from body language. Attend to the volume, pacing, emphasis, intensity, emotive quality, and also what is *not* said. Be alert to body language, nuances of expression, and the feeling level during this type of conversation.

Sensitive manual exploration of the presenting painful or tight areas confirms more precisely where problematic areas are located. As you palpate, be sure to evaluate:

• The thickness of the soft tissue
• Its ability to yield
• Localized temperature
• The texture of the skin and underlying tissue
• The range and quality of joint motion

Analyzing the client

After perceiving the client as fully as possible, thoughtful analysis is appropriate. Perform functional testing to reveal injured or compromised structures requiring sculpting and other therapeutic techniques. Both Stanley Hoppenfeld's classic text, *Physical Examination of the Spine and Extremities*,[1] and the videos and writing of Ben Benjamin, Ph.D.,[2] are clear, comprehensive sources of these types of assessment procedures. Identify any causative factors listed in Chapter Three, and consult and/or refer to physicians for medical treatment if indicated. Note adaptations or contraindications that are appropriate for your client, and plan your work accordingly.

Your careful analysis can answer the following relevant questions:

• What structures comprise the tense and/or painful areas?
• Which muscles would be involved in an observable decrease in range of motion?
• Which muscles are involved in producing an observed habitual movement pattern, such as swinging one hip into external rotation when walking?
• If there are postural imbalances, such as tilting the head to one side or excessive lumbar lordosis, what structures are involved in maintaining that imbalance?
• What tissue needs to be lengthened to balance muscle pairs, and what needs to be strengthened and toned?
• Are there any conditions that would contraindicate sculpting or necessitate caution in working with this client?
• What areas of the body might harbor the fears or emotional charges revealed by the client?
• Are there any limitations in positioning on the table to consider, such as pregnancy, casting, or recent surgery?

Intuiting the needs of the client: a three-centers approach

In many traditional schema of body energies, humans are seen as having instinctive energy centers that guide the physical/emotional functions of the body.

You can use these instincts to more holistically intuit information about a client. Naturally, the more clarity and balance that exist for you in these centers, the more accurate and balanced will be your intuitive powers. By tuning in to your client before, during, and after a session, you can receive input from the yin, feminine, right brain side of yourself to complement the left brain information your analysis has produced.[3]

The body's physical center attends to the sense of personal identity, the conservation and development of the individual's life force, and the body's functioning. This center, that is known variously as the Hara, tan tien, the Manipura chakra, or the physical center, is located three finger-widths below the navel and directly in the middle of the lower abdomen.[4] When questioned directly, your physical center can give intuitive answers to identify the client and her needs. **(Image 11)**

The emotional or heart center, also called the Anahata chakra, is located in the middle of the chest.[5] It attends to the feelings, the sense of relationship, and the impulses and desires of the being. You can look to this center for an intuitive sense of the client's feelings. You can attune your heart center to hear the client's wants. Empathize with this center so that you feel into the client's emotions.

With the intellectual or head center, the Ajna chakra, you can intuitively synthesize the messages from your other senses to produce an image of the intended goal of your work. This center is involved in heightened self-awareness and clear intellectual functioning.[6] It answers the question, "What is happening here?" It accesses the anatomy, physiology, pathology, and kinesiology you understand, and applies this knowledge appropriately to the situation. This sense can guide you to work that fits with the individual and her needs as well as the environment, the time frame, and your own skill level.

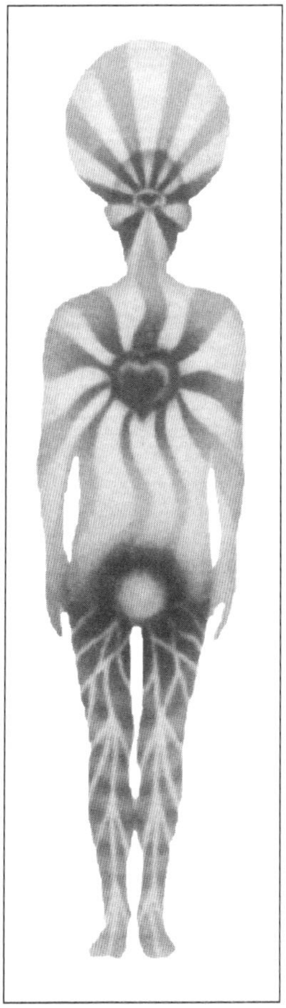

• **Image 11:** *Physical, emotional, and mental concentrations of energy coalesce into instinctive body centers.*

Clarifying then Visualizing Intention

Observation, analysis, and intuition produce a knowledge of what work will be appropriate. Deep tissue sculpting and all bodywork can affect the client posturally, imagistically, archetypally, emotionally, intellectually, physiologically, and spiritually. First, you must synthesize your observations, analysis, and intuitive instincts in answering the question, "What is the effect I want to create?" Then you need to hold this intention in your mind. By focusing on an image, phrase, or sound that carries the sense of your intention, you can more easily and directly enhance your chances of creating that effect. Like the sculptor at his art, hold a mental picture of your intended creation to guide your molding, shaping, and reforming movements as you sculpt.

For example, you may feel that the client's neck needs to be more elongated and her shoulders dropped down and away from her ears. By envisioning this effect as you sculpt, you guide that effect to occur. You also may invite the client to actively imagine this realignment by thinking of her neck and everything behind her ears getting longer while her shoulders drop toward her feet. Metaphorical visualizations such as imagining her neck to be like a plant reaching toward the sun when she is standing, are often effective. Active visualization employs the client's intention to augment the myofascial changes being prompted by your hands.

Body Mechanics

With the functions of observation, analysis, intuition, and imagination completed, you are almost ready to touch the client's body. First, however, you must organize your own body and choose tools to perform the techniques of the method with grace, strength, efficiency, minimal strain to yourself, and minimal pain to your client.

Practitioner's alignment

The ancient Oriental martial art of tai chi chuan teaches many principles that are directly applicable to all bodywork methods, particularly the deep tissue styles.[7] Upright posture with bipolar extension into the head and down toward the earth is fundamental. All of your movements must originate in the tan tein, the physical center, and flow into the relaxed torso through the heart center and into the hands. **(Image 12)** Pressure and momentum for techniques comes from shifting of your weight from your lower body into the client's body. All of your joints are maintained in open, stabilized, and relaxed positions. You should relax and slow your breath, allowing it to originate from deep within your lower abdomen and expand and contract the torso in all directions. (See Chapter Six, pp. 67-70.)

Sculpting tools

Your choice of sculpting tools affects your body position at the table. Any bony body part is a possible tool for you. The

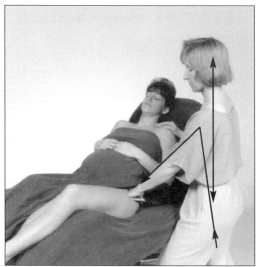

• **Image 12**: *Structural alignment and lean into the client create penetrating, gentle pressure without practitioner injury.*

most commonly used are the fingertips, knuckles and heel of the hand, forearm, and elbow. The smaller and more pointed the tool, the more penetrating and specific its effect on the client's tissue. These smaller tools are best for thin and small muscles and specific sites of tissue disorganization. They are also often the most painful tools for the client. Broader tools, such as the forearm and the fisted hand, deliver more generalized, broader effect to larger areas of tissue. They tend to be less penetrating, may be less painful, and can deliver deepest pressures.

The deeper the structure lies in the client's body, the more pressure that usually will be needed to touch it. Generally, the elbow, forearm, fist and knuckles are better structured to support heavier pressure without risking damage to the practitioner's body. (See Chapter Six, pp. 70-71.)

Technique Types and Applications

There are basically two techniques in deep tissue sculpting: the compression and the compression-to-stroke.

Compression

A compression occurs when the practitioner applies pressure straight into the client's tissue and no movement results, other than deeper into the body. For example, if your elbow is the tool being used, you will first make gentle contact with your elbow only on the skin. If you feel resistance at the skin level, apply no more pressure until that resistance dissolves. The tissue must invite you deeper, or you may sense that

no further depth is possible without creating pain and/or more resistance in the client's body.

By waiting at this first layer of resistance, the client's tissues are "warmed," softening and opening to your pressure. Inducing this change is especially important since you will perform most sculpting prior to applying oil. In other words, there will be no gradually increasing and warming effects such as are generally created by effluerage, kneading, and other Swedish massage therapy techniques. Also, remember the biomechanical properties of connective tissue discussed in Chapter Two; these realities necessitate a passage of up to 30-60 seconds for myofascial tissues to melt under your touch.

This slow, sensitive entrance into the body can be facilitated by utilizing both your own and your client's breath. During an exhale the client may be more receptive to your touch, as exhaling is an emptying movement. Your exhale can be used, perhaps only figuratively, as a momentum to pour your energy into the client's body as your breath outpours.

If the tissue melts, allowing deeper pressure, allow your elbow to sink deeper. You may encounter several layers of resistance and then release. Continue through the layers to the level of the structure that you are intending to touch. That may be the superficial fascia or the muscle beneath, or perhaps the bone that is deepest yet. Always, however, the client is respected and never forced, only coaxed, into opening and relaxing. Feedback from the client using the number or color scale of perceived level of intensity helps in sustaining this correct depth and speed.(See Chapter Two, pp. 28-29 for detailed descriptions of these feedback systems.)

Compression-to-stroke/follow

When you direct your pressure parallel to the muscle fibers being sculpted as well as into the client's tissue, you will likely induce a response that also strokes, elongates, and stretches the muscle and fascia. This compression-to-stroke proceeds, as does the compression, only to the depth, distance, and speed that the client's release allows and no deeper, longer, or faster. There should never be an experience of pushing, pulling, or tearing through the tissue. **(Image 13)**

You should not insist that a muscle be stroked from one end to the other once a stroke is begun, or that it must be compressed for its entire length; that just may not be the way the fascia gives. What usually happens is that a muscle will release in such a way that some compressions and some compression-to-stroke techniques will happen. Since the yielding of the client determines the technique, any combination or sequence is possible. You can only intend a particular effect, position your body to facilitate that happening, and then respond to what actually happens.

Working Without Oil

While many types of massage therapy use oil to reduce friction, deep tissue sculpting usually does not. With oil on the skin, the speed of the work will follow

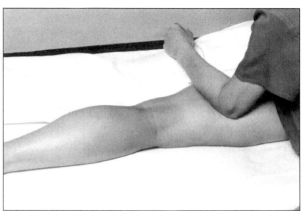

• **Image 13**: *Tissue yield should create any sculpting movement on the skin.*

the slipperiness of the skin rather than the deeper tissues' yielding. The structures to be sculpted are below skin level so sliding on the skin will not create the desired result. Of course, if either the client's or your skin is extremely dry or clammy, a very small amount of light oil, lotion, or cocoa butter might be appropriate on your hands or forearm. Using oil very sparingly on the hair should also alleviate painful pulling on very hairy areas of the chest, back, or legs. When integrated with Swedish, other circulatory massage, or other lubricant assisted methods, perform sculpting first or remove excess oil before sculpting.

Targeting and Completing Techniques

Whichever technique is used, you must choose where, precisely, to apply a technique. Compressing directly into the center or vortex of the holding pattern of the tissue is often very effective in eliciting myofascial release. Sometimes, however, working first with the surrounding tissue better contacts the problematic area. Neighboring muscles that are involved may need to be relaxed initially, or perhaps working superior or inferior to particularly tight and sensitive spots will provide a "back door" entrance into the tension vortex.

A particular technique is completed when the client cannot release any further, when the intended effect has been accomplished, or when you can no longer sustain that particular compression or stroke. Exit is made with the same sensitivity to the client's response as was followed in entering. Release your pressure slowly at a speed that allows the tissue to adjust to your change in pressure and to maintain the tissue stretch and elongation that has occurred. If you want to attempt further release, choose a new positioning or tool, then proceed. Enhance the circulatory effects of sculpting at this time with techniques such as effleurage and kneading strokes. Reinforce alignment and perceptual changes with passive joint movement integrated after sculpting techniques.

Receptivity and Responsiveness: A Three-Centers Approach

The previous sections have been exploring the mechanical and physical aspects of deep tissue sculpting. From a three-centers point of view, the body mechanics, choice of tools, and types of techniques are all aspects governed from the physical center. For effective somatic bodywork, however, the practitioner also must utilize his emotional and intellectual centers in performing a technique.

When you engage your emotional center,

you tap into your nurturing, loving side. You can feel empathy with your client's feelings and state of being. You work with respect for limitations, releases, and resistances without indulging the client's or your own overly sentimental responses. On the other hand, you should not be rigidly insensitive to feelings, proceeding on with technique regardless of the client's response. Allow a sense of unity, or what the creator of psychophysical integration, the late Milton Trager, M.D., called "hookup,"[8] to develop. In that state, the connection between the client and you is profound. (See Chapter Four, pp. 50-53.)

The intellectual center engages in sculpting when the mind is emptied of all thoughts except those focused on the work at hand. If you focus on a phrase or visualization, such as the phrase "drop the shoulders" or the word "melting" repeated over and over, other extraneous ideas usually float away. Without the usual clutter and chatter of the mind, the intellect then is freer and more open to insights that occur as the work proceeds. You should not, however, hold rigidly to your original intention in the face of new information and understanding. Use intention as a beginning place and as a comparison point for new input received from the client.

Clients' Perceptions and Responses

Clients often will experience sensations during deep tissue sculpting similar to those perceived by the practitioner. Tense areas may be felt as hard, tight, impenetrable, and perhaps painful. Sometimes, however, there is numbness in chronically tight areas. When pressure is applied to these areas, the client may have no physical sensation except pressure. When questioned sensitively, some clients notice imagery, symbolism, or metaphors related to their bodily experience. Her tense abdomen can feel like an empty pit, a boiling stew, or just intensely dark and sticky to her. Sometimes these areas will reveal emotional sensations. As she pays attention to the tight spot, she may feel fearful, sad, or angry, and that awareness can intensify and/or resolve with increased pressure.

A client may experience relaxation on a physical level, as a letting go, a stretching sensation, a melting or dissolving sense. Her awareness may be keenly focused on the muscle being worked, and she observes every nuance of change. Movements may begin to occur that further expend the tension. Sometimes it is the client's experience to feel no relaxation sensations.

She may experience warmth or tingling at the site or at distant points. She may feel pain at the point of compression or at some referred site. Often sculpting uncovers myofascial trigger points, hypersensitive soft tissue areas referring pain to sites distant from the touched area.[9] When located, continue to sculpt until these painful neurological referral points are desensitized.

She may be aware of various generalized body responses such as changes in her breathing, trembling, perspiration, or tingling. Lightheadedness sometimes occurs, as does either an overall lightness or heaviness in her body. Sometimes she will be very agitated, especially if emotional expression is blocked. She may feel very meditative, calmed, and serene. Most clients feel profoundly touched and known with deep tissue sculpting.

Summary of Chapter Five

1. As a practitioner of deep tissue sculpting, you must develop skills in understanding your client, in body mechanics, technique, and receptivity and responsiveness.
2. To understand your client and her needs as fully as possible, use all your senses to gather information and your intellect and intuition to analyze it; then engage your imaginal powers to visualize the most appropriate outcome for your client.
3. To gather information, begin by looking at and listening to your client and by feeling the tissues and structures that she has indicated are tense or painful.
4. To help you interpret your client's information, submit it to further analysis based on your knowledge and experience.
5. By using your awareness from your own physical, emotional and mental centers, you can deepen your intuitive understanding of your client's instinctive needs.
6. Ask yourself, "What is the effect I want to achieve?" Then create and hold in your mind's eye the mental image that represents the best response.
7. Before you begin to work, organize your body efficiently and choose the most effective sculpting tools.
8. Organize your body around your physical center, keeping grounded, extended through your spine and open through your upper body. Shift your weight to achieve pressure and momentum, and maintain full, relaxed breathing.
9. Choose as sculpting tools the bony body parts most suited to your positioning at the table, the characteristics of the area you are sculpting, the tissue quality, and the desired effect.
10. Deep tissue sculpting uses two basic techniques, compression and compression-to-stroke/follow. Use and combine them according to the way your client's tissue yields.
11. For a compression, make initial contact with the appropriate tool at the area to be worked, then wait for the tension to melt.
12. For a compression-to-stroke/follow, sink your pressure straight in but also along the direction of the structures so that as the tissue releases, you are invited to stroke and lengthen the muscle and fascia.
13. You will usually sculpt without oil on the skin so as to keep contact with the deeper structures and maintain a slow, even pace prompted by the client's tissues yielding.
14. Sinking into the center of a holding pattern is often the best way to achieve release, but you may sometimes want to release surrounding areas first.
15. When you feel that the tissue has released all that it is going to or that you cannot sustain the technique, slowly and sensitively exit your client's body.
16. You use your three centers during a sculpting session: your physical center to arrange and carry out the session, your emotional center to "hook up" with your client, and your mental center to hone and focus intention.
17. During the sculpting session, your client may experience any amount and intensity of physical sensation and emotion.

Sources Cited

[1] Hoppenfeld, Stanley. *Physical Examination of the Spine and Extremities*. New York, NY: Appleton-Century-Crofts, 1976.

[2] Benjamin, Ben with Gale Borden, M.D. *Listen to Your Pain*. New York, NY: Penguin Books, 1984.

[3] Rose, Colin and Malcolm J. Nicholl. *Accelerated Learning for the 21st Century*. New York, NY: Delacorte Press, 1997, pp.32-35.

[4] Dyctwald, Ken. *Bodymind*. New York, NY: Jove Publications, 1978, pp.118-140.

[5] Dyctwald, Op. Cit. pp.141-182.

[6] Dyctwald, Op. Cit. p.236.

[7] Galante, Lawrence. *Tai Chi: The Supreme Ultimate*. York Beach, ME: Samuel Weiser, 1981, pp.25-27.

[8] Calvert, Robert. "Exclusive Interview with Dr. Milton Trager," *Massage Magazine*, Issue 15, August/September, 1988, pp.12-32.

[9] Chaitow, Leon. *Modern Neuromuscular Techniques*. London, UK: Churchill Livingstone, 1997, p.xi.

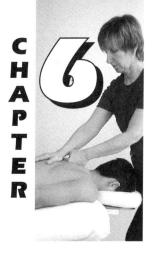

Health Maintenance for the Practitioner's Hands and Body

Care, development, and protection of your hands and body are crucial for effectiveness and career longevity no matter which bodywork or massage specialty you practice. Because of the stress of sustained pressures used in deep tissue work, deep tissue practitioners need to be especially mindful of health maintenance including:

- Balanced alignment of the entire body and appropriate weight shifts to apply pressure
- Appropriate choice and variety of tools utilized, i.e. fingertips, knuckles, elbow, and others
- Extra bracing and specific alignment of the entire pectoral girdle, including the scapulothoracic, shoulder, elbow, wrist, and finger joints
- Increasing dexterity and strength
- Regular cleansing and maintenance

Body Alignment and Weight Shift
Table size and height

Strength, focus, endurance, relaxation, and receptivity in the hands result from effective use of the entire body. Proper table width and height are the first requirements to achieve efficient, stress-free body alignment. A 27"-30"-wide table will usually allow the client adequate room, while enabling most practitioners to shift their weight over the table without excessive leaning and strain to their backs. Choose a narrower table if you are short; however, you will then need sidearms or some other measures to accommodate larger client's arms.

Most practitioners work best with their table height adjusted so that, when standing erect, the tabletop touches between fingertips and wrist when the arm hangs loosely at the side. This height encourages and allows for use of the lower body for pressure and weight shifting without extreme knee bends or muscling technique from the upper body. Of course, if you have unusual body proportions, modify this rule of thumb to your body shape. When working with side-lying clients, the higher end of this range allows for the more horizontal weight shift involved. Adapt to heavier clients and when using a contoured bodyCushion® or other client positioners with table settings at the lower end of this range.

Stance and weight shift

When standing beside a massage table, plant your feet firmly on the floor, usually your shoulders' width apart and with one foot ahead of the other by one to three foot lengths. Flex your knees. Don't tire yourself with too deep a stance, but avoid limiting your weight shift and maneuverability with too shallow a stance. You can shift your body weight directly into your working tool if your torso is facing toward the point where you intend to apply pressure. The more direct the vector of pressure applied the less energy required to achieve effective depth. Think of the physical center (tan tein) as a flashlight pointing the way, and aim it as directly as possible at the structure you want to sculpt.

In fact, aligning your spine, with no twists, rotations, or excessive curvatures, especially of the lumbar and cervical areas, is crucial in minimizing stress and avoiding injury. Lengthen your entire spine, but maintain gentle curvatures. To get lower, bend at your hip joints or knees and not from your waist, which can strain your lower back. Notice and correct any collapse or sidebending of your head or torso. Look downward when you need to locate structures and monitor client reaction, then realign your head on your spine, reestablishing a gentle cervical curvature with your chin gently tucked in. **(Image 14)**

With balanced alignment, and the table at the proper size and height, you are ready to perform your technique, whether it will be a slow, melting deep tissue sculpt, an effleurage, a knead, a compression into a trigger point, or a passive joint movement. Gather your weight into your rear leg, emptying your front leg of weight but allowing it to remain relaxed, resting on the floor. Initiate and maintain momentum by pushing into the ground with the rear leg, but do not lock your knee in doing so. Direct your weight into your working tool, and avoid loading your front leg, which should remain empty, relaxed, and free to step if needed. Increase pressure by pressing into the ground to lean more heavily onto your tool, and lighten it by shifting subtly back into the rear leg. Release your pressure by regathering your weight into the rear leg. With each technique applied, push from the back leg

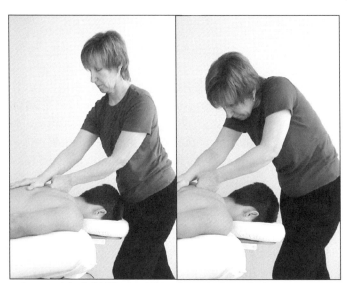

• **Image 14**: *(left) Weight shifting from the lower body is more efficient and comfortable. (right) Upper body "muscling" of technique usually creates pectoral girdle and spinal collapse and pain.*

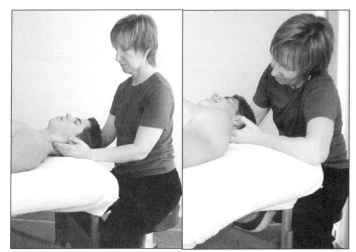

• **Image 15**: *Effective body use involves (left) relaxed, erect alignment. (right) Sustained sidebending of either head or torso can create both practitioner and client pain.*

into the area being compressed or stroked. Accomplish movements away from the client's body, such as many traction stretches and return effleurage, by similarly shifting weight from front foot to back foot.

For procedures that require you to squarely face the side of the table, such as petrissage or some lomi-lomi strokes, a "horse riding" stance is more efficient. In this stance, your feet are parallel to each other, at least as far apart as your shoulders' width, and your knees are flexed. Weight shifting between the feet should power your arms for techniques.

In a seated position, plant your feet firmly on the floor. In this position, the actual weight shifts must result from your ischial tuberosities pressing into the stool or chair, thereby, functioning as the feet do when standing. Of course, always maintain spinal alignment with the head erect, and relax your shoulder girdle. **(Image 15)**

Upper body alignment

Relax all unnecessary contraction of the pectoral girdle muscles so that your shoulders remain down, balanced on the torso, and relaxed. Avoid hunching and anterior rounding of the shoulders when applying techniques. Your deltoids, pectoralis major, biceps, triceps, latissimus dorsi, and trapezius will not be overused if you use your body weight efficiently to create pressure rather than push from your arms. To stabilize your shoulder and scapulothoracic joints as you shift your weight into your client's body, balance the functions of the serratus anterior/ rhomboids, the latissimus dorsi/upper trapezius, along with the humeral stabilizers, i.e., teres minor, infraspinatus, and subscapularis. Proper care of your shoulder and scapulothoracic joints while working avoids injuries such as rotator cuff syndrome, shoulder bursitis, muscular strain, and kyphosis.

When the forearm or elbow is used in deep tissue bodywork, only the contraction of the elbow flexors is necessary; keep the forearm, wrist, and hand relaxed. Stabilize the shoulder and scapulothoracic joints in an open, balanced position avoiding excessive humeral adduction or abduction, and let your shifted body weight be the source of pressure. Apply no pressure from the other hand, the head, or the shoulder and back muscles. This will avoid strain to your upper extremity. You will also prevent possible injuries such as

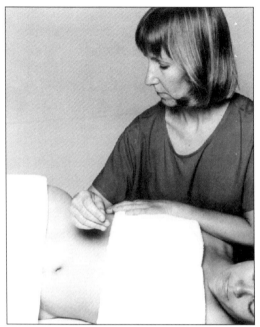

• **Image 16**: *Relaxed shoulder, arm and hand positions deliver deep, sensitive sculpting.*

cervical strain and misalignment, bursitis, rotator cuff syndrome, tennis elbow and neuritis. **(Image 16)**

Joint Protection

Your hands perceive the needs of the tissue beneath. They perform fine, delicate movements as they direct energy and apply appropriate technique. They sustain the weight of the your body as you apply compressions, stroking, or kneading procedures. They are the most important tools of your trade.

You must protect the integrity of your fingers, wrists, and elbows. Whatever technique you apply, perform it with as much open, balanced alignment of the joints as possible. If you repeatedly hyperextend your wrist joint during deep palmar and hypothenar strokes, carpal

tunnel syndrome, tendonitis, and/or ligament strain in the wrist can result. Excessive pressure on your fingertips, particularly the thumb, can hyperextend or hyperflex the metacarpal-phalangeal joint. The resulting ligament strain and stretching can cause pain, swelling, and instability in the affected joints. Brace or support your fingers and hands to create additional protection for the joints sustaining the greatest pressures. For example, the fisted hand can brace your thumb, or your other hand can act as a splint for the phalangeal joints when fingertip pressure is required.

Exclusive and/or improper use of any tool, but especially the thumbs, the heel of the hand, or the fingertips, can result in joint-structure damage. Reserve these tools for small areas, for thinner, less tense muscles, and for specific, definition-type work. By regularly using alternative tools such as your knuckles, forearm, and elbows, you can sensitize them to nearly as fine a receptivity as your fingertips. Since the structure of the elbow and fisted hand are more capable of sustaining deep

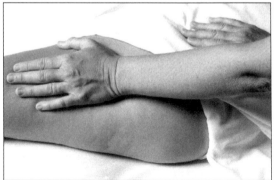

• **Image 17**: *Avoiding wrist hyperextension and overuse of the heel of the hand prevents painful wrist syndromes.*

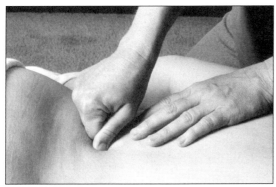

• **Image 18**: *Thumbs are more protected when used sparingly and braced.*

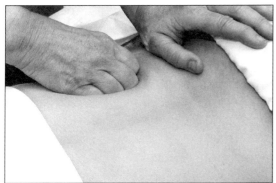

• **Image 19**: *Knuckles penetrate deeply yet softly if hand and forearm remain relaxed.*

pressure without threat to joint integrity, use these tools for deepest pressures whenever possible. Irritation and inflammation of the joint capsule, strained ligaments, osteoarthritis, and carpal tunnel syndrome are all probable results of using one tool more than others, or attempting to release large masses of muscle with smaller tools such as thumbs or fingertips. **(Images 17,18,19)**

Developing Strength
Hands and pectoral girdle

Work with both left and right sides of your body so that one hand and arm will not be less strong or agile than the other.

You can increase strength, control, and dexterity in your hands while enjoying the products and pleasures of typing, weed pulling, or playing piano, guitar, or rhythm instruments. Other more structured exercises include:

- Squeezing a firm ball, such as a tennis ball, or a product available in many athletic stores called Power Putty™
- Touching each fingertip to thumbtip in a smooth, increasingly brisk rhythm
- Fisting your hand, then rhythmically squeezing it tighter, moving from little finger, to ring finger, and so on through the thumb, and repeating this sequence increasingly faster and for more repetitions as the hand develops
- Pushing the fingertips of one hand against those of the other, either simultaneously, or from little finger through thumb in a rhythmic sequence
- Rhythmically rolling three marbles or large steel ball bearings in your palm
- Placing a poker chip between two fingers and "walking" it to the next two fingers and back without using the other hand
- Playing tossing games with first one poker chip then as many as three, developing both one -and two-handed tossing and catching patterns

Proper alignment and balance of your pectoral girdle as it sustains much of your body weight is difficult without adequate upper body strength. Maintain a regular program of weight training, exercise, or other activities that target strength and flexibility in these muscles: biceps, triceps, shoulder joint stabilizers, latissimus dorsi, trapezius, rhomboids, and, most importantly, the serratus anterior. The serratus provide critical downward rotation of the scapula, stabilizing it and the rest of your shoulder girdle against the posterior driving force you create when leaning your body weight to sculpt.

Most practitioners can easily incorporate daily push-ups to develop a foundation of pectoral girdle strength. If you cannot do a full push-up, then work towards that goal with progressively more strenuous push-up variations. Start by doing pushaways:

1. Stand one to two feet from a wall or other sturdy flat vertical surface.
2. Place your palms or your fisted knuckles against the wall and lean onto them while sustaining a rigid position.
3. Drop toward and then push your upper body away from the wall, maintaining alignment of your scapula against your back.
4. Repeat for 12 repetitions, rest and repeat 12 times. After several weeks of regular exercise, intensify the effort required by standing further and further from the wall, thereby taking more and more of your body weight onto your arms.
5. Progress to the floor push-ups when you feel ready. Initially, hold your weight on your knees and hands, moving to standard military push-ups on toes and hands when your strength is sufficiently developed.

Increasing overall body energy: a tai chi exercise

Protect and strengthen your hands by increasing overall body energy and by learning to direct that energy through your hands. Traditional Oriental disciplines such as tai chi chuan and Chi Gung are notable for their effect in developing the body's vital energy (the Chi). If experienced teachers in these arts are unavailable, video instruction can be helpful.[1] The following basic exercise from tai chi done daily is also recommended:

1. Stand with your feet at your shoulders' width apart and with your feet directly under your shoulders. Distribute your weight evenly between both feet and throughout each foot.
2. Achieve a relaxed, bipolar extension of your spine—imagine a string attached to the crown of your head extending your spine upward toward the sky; at the same time, imagine a weight at your coccyx extending your spine downward toward the earth. Let your arms hang loosely at your sides.
3. Maintain this upright and extended alignment of your spine throughout the exercise.
4. Gradually bend into your knees. Step straight ahead with your left foot, placing it, with the toes pointing straight ahead, one or two foot-lengths ahead of the right. Shift 70% of your weight forward into your left foot. Turn the toes of your right foot outward to a 45° angle. Your torso should be facing ahead. (This position is called the Bow Stance in tai chi and is recommended above as your

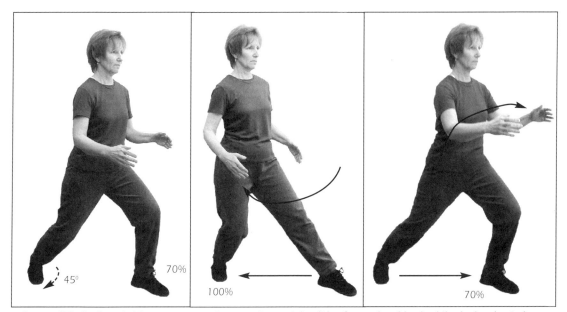

• **Image 20**: *In the tai chi energy generation exercise, weight slides forward and back while the hands circle.*

initial stance at tableside.)

5. Bend your arms at the elbows to a 90⁰ angle, and let your palms face each other as if holding a beach ball in front of your abdomen. Relax any shoulder tension. **(Image 20, left)**

6. As you gradually shift 100% of your weight back into your right leg, begin creating a circle in front of your abdomen by moving your arms down and back. Inhale gently and fully from your lower abdomen. **(Image 20, center)**

7. As you gradually shift your weight forward 70% into your left leg, continue the circular movement of your arms up and forward. Exhale gently and fully from your lower abdomen. The full circle of your arms also will be about beach ball size. **(Image 20, right)**

8. Continue the slow, coordinated movement of your weight and torso with the circular movement of your arms for 2-5 minutes.

9. Repeat the exercise with your right foot forward.

Regular Maintenance

As you already know, clip and file your nails regularly, and keep your hands clean, smooth, and free of calluses and rough spots. Protect your hands with gloves when gardening, using harsh cleaners, or doing manual labor. In addition, self-massage of your hands is invaluable for keeping them tension-free. Use deep, melting compressions of the muscles down to the bone; eliminate trigger points; and wring and strip any accumulated tension from your hands and forearms daily or, at least, weekly. Use post-event sports massage techniques for any stressed areas of the pectoral girdle, arms, or hands. Increase and clarify energy flow in your hands by regularly and systematically sculpting and stripping each fingertip, including anterior, posterior, and nail surfaces.

Attentive care of your hands is as crucial for effectiveness and vitality of your trade as is advanced or specialized skill enhancement. Avoid debilitating injuries and discomfort by proper body alignment, extra support for your joints, increasing pectoral girdle and hand strength, using a variety of tools, and regularly maintaining your hands.

Summary of Chapter Six

1. Proper body alignment, efficient weight shifting, and protection of your hands and other sculpting tools will help prevent injury and strain and contribute to your effectiveness and career longevity.
2. Appropriate table height and width help you maintain efficient, stress-free body alignment as you work.
3. You work most effectively at the table when your lower body is the solid base of support that moves your weight into your sculpting tool, your spine is lifted through the top of your head and organized around its natural curvatures, and your torso is aimed toward the structure you are sculpting.
4. Standing at the table in a tai chi Bow Stance or a "horse riding" stance allows you to shift your weight to support the specific work of your hands and other sculpting tools. In a seated position, your weight shifting is accomplished through your ischial tuberosities.
5. To prevent overuse of your hands and upper body, stabilize the muscles of your pectoral girdle so that your weight can pour through it into your sculpting tool and the client's body.
6. To protect your joints while working, keep them open, aligned and supported, select the proper tool for the area to be released, and develop effective alternative tools to avoid overuse.
7. Improve the strength and dexterity of your hands through both regular activities and more structured exercise. Develop strength and stability in your pectoral girdle through a weight program or exercises like push-ups or pushaways.
8. On a daily basis, practice exercises like those from Oriental disciplines that increase your body's overall vitality and direct its flow into your hands.
9. Taking care of your hands through regular grooming, self-massage and appropriate protection helps you maintain the effectiveness of your work and prevent injury and discomfort.

Sources Cited

[1] "T'ai Chi for Health" (video). Venice, CA: Healing Arts Publishing Inc., 800-2-LIVING.

ACCOMPLISHING

- Deep Tissue Sculpting Session for the Back
- Deep Tissue Sculpting Session for the Low Back and Abdomen
- Deep Tissue Sculpting Session for the Neck and Shoulders
- Full Body Sculpting and Applications to Other Body Areas

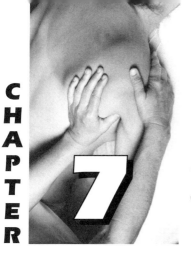

7

Deep Tissue Sculpting Session for the Back

The human back is constructed of amazingly overlapped layers of muscles and fascial sheets. This soft tissue surrounds the spinal core creating uprightness and flexibility, and generating the mechanical dynamics of breathing. It cloaks the middle and upper back with a drapery of muscles allowing for both graceful and powerful expression through the arms and hands. Muscle and fascial bands connect the torso to the supporting earth through the legs.

Unfortunately, however, the elegantly designed back is all too commonly the site of generalized tension, taut, ropy muscles, and painfully stiff joints that limit its inherent potential. The techniques that follow in this chapter begin the process of opening up the more superficial and middle layers of the back. Because of its relationship with both the pectoral and pelvic girdle, this session will necessarily include work opening these areas. While it is limited to posterior structures, this session can be augmented with anterior procedures detailed in later chapters. Thc more core structures (especially quadratus lumborum and iliopsoas muscles) are also addressed there.(See Chapter Eight, pp. 94-96.)

Guiding Imagery for the Session: Elongate the Back; Open the Pectoral Girdle

The chronically tense client who complains of pain and tension in the upper and midback regions usually will appear to be shortened throughout the extensor muscles and the fascia of the back. Additionally, the pectoral girdle may seem closed and restricted either on the anterior or posterior sides. The shoulder girdle also may appear either depressed, elevated, and/or rotated. Observe and evaluate your client's personal tension patterns.

Remember that you are guiding your work with your intention. For this client, imagine elongating the back and opening the pectoral girdle to facilitate release. Create a mental picture of lengthened spinal extensors, pliable posterior fascial planes, and relaxed pectoral muscles as the overall theme or intention around which the following detailed procedures can evolve. Hold these images as pictures in your mind's eye (and sometimes ask your client to imagine the same) as you sculpt these areas.

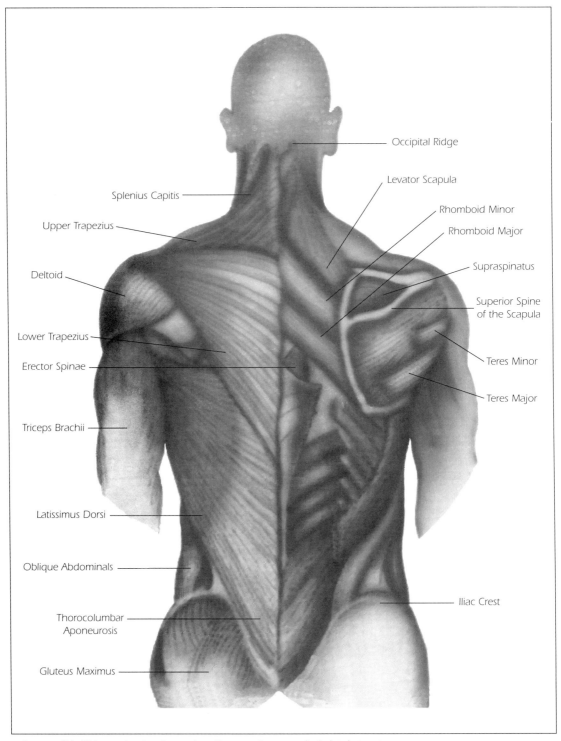

- Occipital Ridge

- Levator Scapula

- Rhomboid Minor

- Rhomboid Major

- Supraspinatus

- Superior Spine of the Scapula

- Teres Minor

- Teres Major

- Iliac Crest

Splenius Capitis

Upper Trapezius

Deltoid

Lower Trapezius

Erector Spinae

Triceps Brachii

Latissimus Dorsi

Oblique Abdominals

Thorocolumbar Aponeurosis

Gluteus Maximus

• **Image 21**: *This session involves primarily posterior musculoskeletal structures.*

General Guidelines

Open your session with contact and evaluation techniques. The procedures detailed below are all designed to facilitate elongation of the back and opening of the pectoral girdle. Observation and evaluation of your individual client should guide you in determining which of these are appropriate and most effective for that client; some might be omitted, and others might be emphasized as discussed at the end of these procedures.

Augment your sculpting with sequences from other modalities, and include movement or stretches that further your intention and provide transition, and that are uniquely created for your individual client. There are other types of soft tissue therapies that you might integrate into these procedures or blend together to further enhance their effect. Bring closure to your work with techniques that integrate the remainder of your client's body.

Several of these sculpting techniques may also be effective as part of a primarily circulatory or passive movement massage session, for example. Create and integrate sculpting as part of an eclectic bodywork approach to the individuals with whom you work. (See also Chapter Eleven: pp. 117-136.)

Sculpting Procedures

The following techniques are described for the client in prone or sidelying position. Use elbow, forearm, fist, knuckle, or finger, depending on your client's and your relative sizes and the depth of structure to be sculpted. Dashed lines on photos represent areas to sculpt; solid arrows denote vector of pressure to apply.

1. Upper trapezius (Image 22)

Intention and imagery: To elongate the upper trapezius myofascia across the shoulders, thereby allowing the shoulders to drop and broaden.

Procedure: Compress and/or stroke the trapezius from near the neck to the acromioclavicular joint.

Hints:

1. Do not use so deep a compression as to "bump" over the deeper-lying muscles.

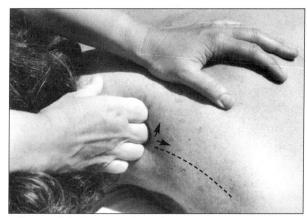

• **Image 22**: *Use a broad tool for the upper trapezius.*

2. You may sculpt both sides simultaneously, or work with one side at a time.

2. Superior spine of the scapula (Image 23)

Intention and imagery: To increase skeletal awareness of the scapula and to relax the trapezius and supraspinatus attachments on the spine of the scapula, thereby allowing the shoulders to drop and broaden.

Procedure: Compress and/or stroke along the superior edge of the spine of the scapula, moving laterally out to the acromioclavicular joint. Sculpt both sides simultaneously, or work with one side at a time.

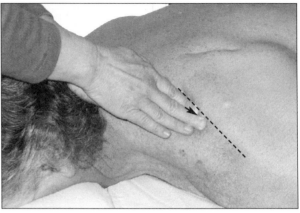

• **Image 23**: *Use a small, pointed tool for spine of scapula attachments.*

3. Lower trapezius (Image 24)

Intention and imagery: To elongate the lower trapezius fibers and the associated deep fascia, releasing the scapula to a more balanced position.

Procedure: Sculpt along the lateral "free" edge of the trapezius, elongating the fibers where glued and bunched to the underlying fascia and muscles. Begin near the upper vertebral border of the scapula and continue toward T-12.

Hints:

1. Remember that the trapezius is a superficial muscle. Avoid "bumping" over the underlying muscles, whose fibers run in directions different than the trapezius. Keep your focus and depth of pressure specifically on the trapezius. Do not push against unyielding tissue in order to force a stroke to happen; a series of compressions along this edge is just as effective.

2. If you have difficulty locating the free edge of the trapezius, find the medial end of the spine of the scapula and T-12, and then draw an imaginary line between these two points to approximate the location of the trapezius.

3. You may want to sculpt multidirectionally at the intersection of the trapezius, rhomboid major, erector spinae, and latissimus dorsi where there will often be a knot of disorganized fascia.

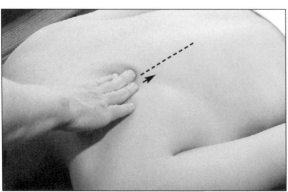

• **Image 24**: *Angle your pressure to "skim" beneath the skin and adipose layers to sculpt the lower trapezius.*

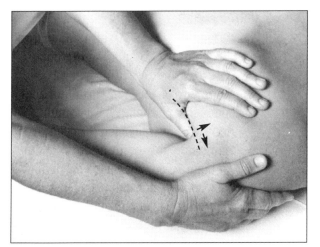

• **Image 25**: *Support the pectoral girdle from elevation when sculpting the teres muscles.*

4. Teres major and minor (Image 25)

Intention and imagery: To relax tension in the teres muscles and open the posterior axillary fascia.

Procedure:

1. Open the the teres muscles along the lateral border of the scapula with compressions beginning near the inferior angle of the scapula.

2. Release the bellies of the two muscles and the accompanying fascia with a compression into the "V" formed by the teres minor and the deltoid.

3. Release the insertion of the teres minor by compressing under the deltoid to the greater tubercle of the humerus.

4. Release the insertion of the teres major with a compression under the deltoid to the bicipital groove of the humerus.

5. Rhomboids (Image 26)

Intention and imagery:

1. To elongate and relax the rhomboid myofascia to allow the scapulae to assume a more balanced position on the ribcage.

2. To bring awareness to the rhomboids.

Procedure:

1. Begin compressing the rhomboid minor from near C-7 toward the insertion on the root of the spine of the scapula and along the vertebral border.

2. Repeat similar sculpts to the rhomboid major, the final sculpt beginning near T-5.

Hints:

1. Precise focus and depth of pressure will be required to avoid bumping over the erector spinae muscles.

2. If the scapula is very rigidly glued to the ribcage, compressions along the vertebral scapula border might be more effective

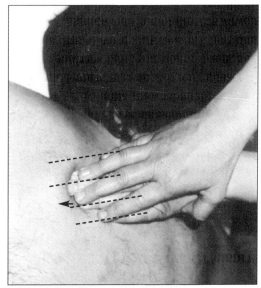

• **Image 26**: *Fingertips work well on smaller clients; bulkier rhomboids may require elbows.*

initially, or it may be more effective to first release the rhomboid major.

3. Underdeveloped rhomboids are common in individuals with "winged" scapulae. Bringing awareness to these muscles so that appropriate toning can be suggested will be a more primary need for these clients.

6. Lengthening the back (Image 27)

<u>Intention and imagery</u>: To elongate and relax the muscles and fascia attaching to and paralleling the spine, primarily trapezius, rhomboids, erector spinae, and posterior fascial sheaths.

<u>Procedure</u>: From a position in front of the client's head, begin stroking/compressing along the tissue lateral to the spine. Continue from near the C-7 area to base of the sacrum, changing tools as the muscles narrow above and over the sacrum.

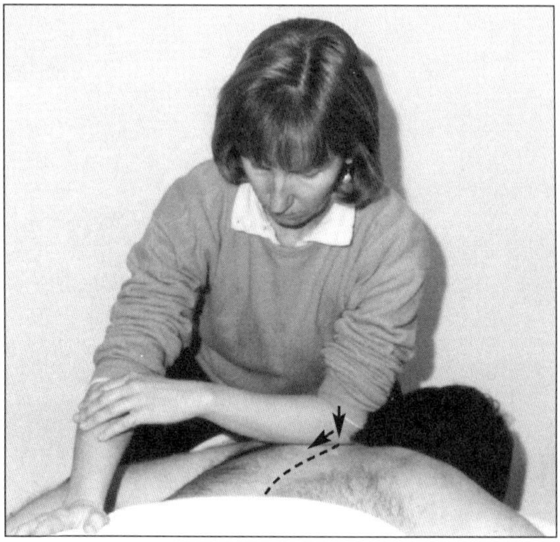

<u>Precaution</u>:

1. Do not stroke directly over spinous processes, but instead apply pressure lateral of them.

• **Image 27**: *Lengthen the back by waiting for tissue to yield, and/or doing a series of compressions.*

2. In the lumbar area, be sure to direct pressure more toward the sacrum than toward the anterior to avoid excessively curving the lower back.

3. If lumbar lordosis is extreme, support the area with a small pillow beneath the abdomen, or do this and all other prone procedures with the client sidelying on her back.

<u>Hints</u>:

1. You may work both sides simultaneously, or left then right sides of the back.

2. On this and on all sculpting procedures, do not force an unbroken stroke if the tissue is not elongating. A series of compressions is equally as effective, and a combination of strokes and compressions will more likely be the release pattern.

3. Change tools as needed to avoid excessive leaning over the table.

7. Vertebra (Image 28)

Intention and imagery:

1. To bring awareness to the individual elements of the spinal column.
2. To release fascia and muscles attaching along the spinous processes of the vertebrae.

Procedure: Using a narrow tool, compress against the side of the spinous process of each vertebra. Make a series of compressions from C-7 down to the sacrum, or follow any elongating movement with a sculpting stroke.

Hints:

1. You may release both sides simultaneously, or sculpt on each side individually.

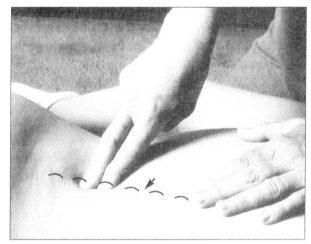

• **Image 28**: *Attachments along the vertebra require more specific tools and less pressure than muscle bellies.*

2. Watch your own alignment to avoid excessive leaning over the table.
3. Avoid excess anterior pressure on the spine especially in the lumbar area.
4. If a face cradle is used so that the neck is straight instead of turned to one side, release the cervical vertebrae as well.

8. Defining the iliac crest (Image 29)

Intention and imagery:

Skeletal awareness of the pelvis at the iliac crest by releasing tension in the attaching muscles and elongating the back.

Procedure: Compress superior to the iliac crest, beginning near the lumbosacral joint and progress lateral making a series of compressions. If the tissue yields sufficiently, melt through and release the thorocolumbar aponeurosis, the erector spinae, the quadratus lumborum, and the transverse and oblique abdominals to make contact with the bone.

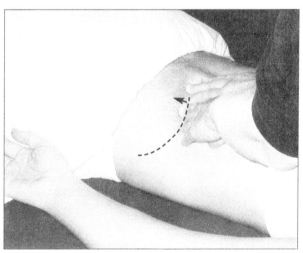

• **Image 29**: *When space is limited, sculpt the superior edge of the iliac crest with fingertips rather than the forearm.*

9. Defining the sacrum and releasing the gluteus (Image 30)

Intention and imagery:
1. Skeletal awareness of the sacrum
2. Elongation of the gluteus maximus myofascia

Procedure:
1. Compress along the border of the sacrum, releasing tension in the attachments of the gluteus maximus to make contact with the bone. Make a series of compressions, moving inferior along the sacrum.
2. Compress and/or stroke the gluteus maximus from origin towards the insertion into the iliotibial tract, elongating and melting the muscle and fascia.

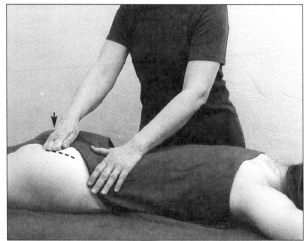

• **Image 30**: *Thick tissue layers of the gluteals require fists or other sturdy tools.*

Precaution:
1. The sciatic nerve is embedded beneath the gluteus maximus and may be sensitive to deep compressions. Change position, direction, or depth of pressure if the client experiences an electrical, burning, numbing, or painful sensation down the posterior of the leg.
2. Be especially sensitive near the coccyx to slowly melt to depth, particularly if there has been any previous injury of the coccyx.

Strokes to Emphasize for Individual Imbalances

Kyphosis

Clients with kyphosis and those with shoulders rounded forward will usually experience more balanced alignment by working the pectoralis major and minor (See Chapter Nine, procedure 7, p. 107.), rectus abdominus (See Chapter Eight, procedure 6, p. 94.), and the rhomboid procedures in this chapter.

Scoliosis

The erector spinae procedure is crucial for scoliosis change, especially working those areas of the muscle within the concave portions of the S-curve of the scoliosis.

Lordosis

Excessive lumbar curvature is addressed in detail with the procedures in Chapter Eight, pp. 87-100.

Pectoral girdle

Upper torso rotations require relaxation of the trapezius, rhomboids, and teres major. Those individuals with shoulders elevated either unilaterally or bilaterally should receive increased attention to the trapezius and levator scapula procedures (See Chapter Nine, procedure 4, pp. 103-104.), while those with retracted, military-stance shoulders require teres minor, trapezius, and rhomboid release.

Supportive Exercise and Stretching

Supplementation of hands-on procedures with movement awareness, stretching, and toning exercise can greatly enhance the sculpting effectiveness. While this manual is not intended to be an exercise book, the following are suggested as supportive activities that your client may use to further facilitate and integrate the effect of the sculpting into her daily activities and awareness.

Movements typical of many African dance patterns involve alternate depression, contraction, and elevation of the ribcage and pectoral girdle. These can be effective movements for establishing balanced function of the paired muscle groups of this area. Done slowly and meditatively, this type of movement also can stretch shortened muscles.

Other stretches, such as a cat stretch done on all fours, and knee-to-chest stretches while lying supine, will also elongate the spinal extensors and the movers and stabilizers of the shoulders. Clasping the arms behind the back will stretch the anterior pectoral muscles. Bob Anderson's popular book *Stretching*[1] details these and other appropriate stretches. Resisting the client's tightening of a tense muscle for five seconds and then taking up the "slack" created when she relaxes that muscle is also effective. Clients may be taught these tense/release exercises to perform throughout their day. Other clients might benefit from the flexibility and body awareness fostered by Feldenkrais based movement exercises such as those explained and illustrated in *Relaxercise*.[2]

Body/Mind Connections

Many psychological theories hold that the body's structure and the way individuals stand, sit, and move within their environments reflect their feelings and beliefs about themselves and their place in the world. As you sculpt the physical tensions of the upper back and shoulders, you might become aware of and address the corresponding emotional tensions. Remember, however, that the client holds her own truth, and that psycholoogical theories are just that—theories.

The whole of the back is often thought to function as though it is a closet where repressed and suppressed feelings are stored and hidden. Typically, the doing and expressing actions of a person are created by the shoulder, arms, hand, and upper back. Specifically, the pectoral girdle often connects the emotional energy of the heart, the breath, and the torso's assimilative centers into the arms and hands and toward vocal expression. Imbalance in these areas can reflect some blockage in the expression of emotion. Shoulders may be rounded forward in a stance of fear and self-protection. They might be rigidly retracted as though to prevent the arms from reaching out in need or compassion, or from striking out in anger. Be aware of the likelihood of emotional aspects of the tight muscles and bunched fascia you are working, and develop your empathy and sensitivity to releasing that tension as well. (See Chapter Four, pp. 48-56.)

Sources Cited

[1] Anderson, Bob. *Stretching*. Bolinas, CA: Shelter Publications Inc., 1980.

[2] Zemach-Bersin, David, Kaethe Zemach-Bersin, and Mark Reese. *Relaxercise*. New York, NY: HarperCollins Publishers, 1990.

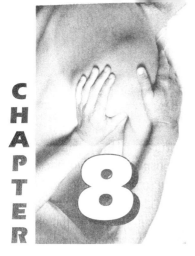

8

Deep Tissue Sculpting Session for the Low Back and Abdomen

Some surveys estimate that 80% of all people will be affected by back pain some time during their lives. For most, this will be primarily low-back pain, as low-back pain ranks second to acute respiratory illness as a cause of time lost from work, according to surveys published in the *Postgraduate Medicine Journal in 1981.*[1] Strains, sprains, damaged or stressed discs, arthritis, and other conditions contribute to and are often at least partially the result of the type of chronic muscle tension that deep tissue sculpting can help reduce.

Because of its frequency and debilitating consequences, some of the more recent massage therapy research has studied the effects of various types of massage therapy on low-back pain.[2] When adults who had experienced low-back pain for at least six months were massaged twice weekly for five weeks for 30 minutes, they experienced a decrease in stress and long-term pain. As compared to a control group who practiced progressive muscle relaxation techniques, the massaged group had less back pain directly after their sessions, fewer depressive symptoms, better sleep, improved range of motion, and an increase in both serotonin and their catecholamine and dopamine biochemical levels—physiological indicators of reduced stress levels.[3]

In a larger trial study of 262 nonspecific, persistent low-back pain sufferers, comparisons of massage therapy, acupuncture and self-care were made. Swedish, deep tissue, and neuromuscular therapy was performed at the discretion of the therapist for up to 10 massages over 10 weeks. Massage appeared to be an effective therapy evidenced by its significant effect on function, reduction in use of pain medications, both short- and long-term benefits, and its lack of significant adverse effects.[4]

Guiding Imagery for the Session
Elongate the Back; Connect the Torso and Legs

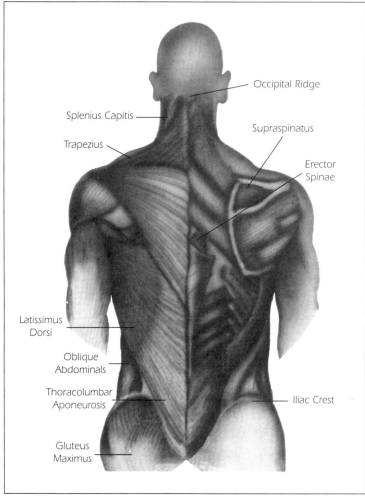

Occipital Ridge

Splenius Capitis

Supraspinatus

Trapezius

Erector Spinae

Latissimus Dorsi

Oblique Abdominals

Thoracolumbar Aponeurosis

Iliac Crest

Gluteus Maximus

• **Image 31**: *Posterior structures are sculpted first in this session.*

Typically, clients complaining of low back pain will present misalignment in the lumbosacral spine, evidenced by excessive curvature or lordosis, flattened lumbar curvature, anterior or posterior tipping of the pelvis, and/or rotations and uneven iliac crest heights. Observe your client's personal tension patterns. His spinal extensor muscles usually will appear as tight, wiry ridges next to the spine, especially in the lumbar area. The lumbodorsal fascia will feel bound to neighboring tissue layers. Relieving the compression of the lumbar spine that is the result of these chronically shortened myofascia is the focus of this session.

Contributing tension in the hamstring group and quadriceps group antagonists and hypotoned or hypertoned abdominals and iliopsoas muscles is also common when there is low-back tension. The client will often appear to be so compacted at the lumbar level that his body's weight does not settle through the pelvis into his legs. It is almost as though his legs are not fully functioning as connectors to the ground, but rather they seem to be as the legs on a stick-man figure. He needs posterior length, anterior to posterior balance, and continuity in function between his torso and lower extremities. This is the other focus of this session.

Inefficient breathing patterns also exacerbate low back pain. Shallow chest breathing and hyperventilating limit the amount and quality of spinal movement. Without the rhythmic waves involved in deep, abdominal expansion during inhalation and full exhalation, the spine can become rigid and inflexible. Because its crural attachments are intimately woven beside the psoas at the anterior lumbar spine, a tense diaphragm can transfer restriction and pain throughout the abdominal and lumbar regions.

Conversely, tension in the lower torso can significantly limit breathing. Abdominal tension can prevent full excursion of the diaphragm by minimizing room available for the necessary displacement of the abdominal organs during inhalation. Other posterior muscles, including the serratus posterior inferior and superior and the levator costarum, influence respiratory depth and ease. When these smaller, more intrinsic muscles are restricted, the ribcage cannot expand to achieve its maximum posterior and lateral excursion.

Direct your work with your intention and an image to hold as your guiding thought while working. For this client, imagine elongating the back, and connecting the torso and legs. Create a mental picture of lengthened spinal extensors and a continuity between the hamstrings and the pelvic myofascia, and between the abdominals and the anterior thigh. Imagine lengthening fluidly through the quadratus lumborum and iliopsoas myofascial connections between the pelvis and the legs. You might also engage your client in imagining elongation and connection as you work together.

General Guidelines

Open your session with contact and evaluation techniques. The procedures detailed below are all designed to facilitate elongation of the back, especially the lumbar area, and the making of connections between the torso and the legs. Observation and evaluation of your individual clients should guide you in determining the appropriateness and efficacy for that client of each of these techniques: some might be omitted, and others might be emphasized, as discussed at the end of these procedures.

Augment your sculpting with sequences from other modalities, and include movement or stretches that further your intention, provide transitions between sculpting, and are uniquely created for your individual client. There are other types of soft tissue therapies that you might integrate into these procedures or blend together to further enhance their effect. Bring closure to your work with techniques that integrate the remainder of your client's body.

Several of these techniques also may be effective as part of a primarily circulatory or passive movement massage session, for example. Create and integrate sculpting as part of an eclectic bodywork approach to the individuals with whom you work. (See Chapter Eleven, pp. 117-136.)

Deep Tissue Sculpting Procedures

The following procedures are to be done with the client prone or sidelying. Use elbow, forearm, fist, knuckle, or finger, depending on your client's and your relative sizes and the depth of structure to be sculpted. Dashed lines on photos represent areas to sculpt; solid arrows denote vector of pressure to apply.

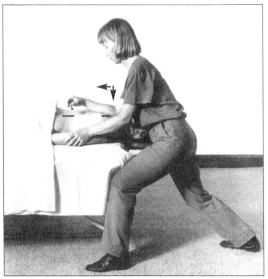

• **Image 32**: *Remember to shift weight from the rear leg to melt into the erector spinae group.*

1. Lengthening the back (Same procedure as in previous session) **(Image 32)**

Intention and imagery: To elongate and relax the muscles and fascia attaching to and paralleling the spine, primarily trapezius, thorocolumbar aponeurosis, rhomboids, erector spinae, and posterior fascial sheaths.

Procedure: From a position in front of the client's head, begin stroking/compressing along the tissue lateral to the spine. Continue from near the C-7 area to base of the sacrum, changing tools as the muscles narrow above and over the sacrum.

Precautions:

1. Do not stroke directly over spinous processes, but instead apply pressure lateral of them.

2. In the lumbar area, be sure to direct pressure more toward the sacrum than anterior to avoid excessively curving the lower back.

3. If lumbar lordosis is extreme, support the area with a folded towel or small pillow beneath the abdomen, or do this and all other prone procedures with the client in a side lying position.

Hints:

1. Work both simultaneously, or left then right sides of the back.

2. As when sculpting any area, do not force an unbroken stroke if the tissue is not elongating. A series of compressions is equally as effective, and a combination of stroking and compressions will more likely be the pattern of release.

3. Change tools as needed to accommodate body position and to avoid excessive leaning over the table.

Procedures 2-4 are to be done first on one side of the body then on the other.

2. Defining the superior and inferior iliac crest (Images 33, 34)

Intention and imagery:

1. Skeletal awareness of the pelvis at the iliac crest by releasing tension in the attaching muscles and fascial sheaths

2. Elongating the back.

Procedure:

1. Compress superior to the iliac crest, beginning near the lumbosacral joint, and progress lateral making a series of compressions. If the tissue yields sufficiently, melt through and

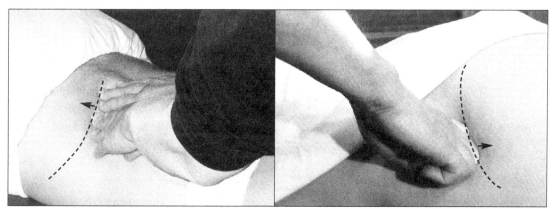

• **Image 33**: *Attachments along the superior edge of the ilium usually require small tools.*   • **Image 34**: *The thicker gluteal attachments on the inferior side call for broader tools.*

release the thorocolumbar aponeurosis, the erector spinae, the quadratus lumborum, and the transverse and oblique abdominals to make contact with the bone. (Same procedure as in previous session.)

2. Compress inferior to the iliac crest, beginning near the lateral side of the posterior iliac spine, and progress lateral making a series of compressions. If the tissue yields sufficiently, melt through and release the attachments of the gluteus medius to make contact with the bone.

3. Defining the sacrum and releasing the gluteal myofascia (Image 35)

Intentions and imagery:

1. Skeletal awareness of the sacrum

2. Elongation of the gluteus maximus myofascia using an image of connecting the torso and the legs

Procedures: (Same procedure as in previous session.)

1. Compress along the lateral border of the sacrum, releasing tension in the attachments of the gluteus maximus to make contact with the bone. Make a series of compressions, moving inferior along the sacrum, to near the coccyx

2. Compress and/or stroke the gluteus maximus from origin toward the insertion into the iliotibial tract, elongating and melting the muscle and fascia.

Precautions:

1. The sciatic nerve is embedded beneath gluteus maximus and may be sensitive to

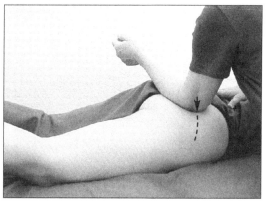

• **Image 35**: *Avoid excess arm and hand tension when using the elbow and forearm for sacrum and gluteal work.*

deep compressions. Change position, direction, or depth of pressure if the client experiences an electrical, burning, numbing, or painful sensation down the posterior of the leg.

2. Be especially sensitive near the coccyx to slowly melt to depth, particularly if there has been any previous injury of the coccyx.

4. Lengthening the hamstring group myofascia (semitendinosis, semimembranosis, biceps femoris) (Image 37)

Intentions and imagery:

1. Elongation of the hamstring muscle group and investing fascia

2. Realignment of the ischial tuberosities from any anterior displacement.

Procedures:

1. Begin with a compression on the ischial tuberosity. Continue with a series of compressions or a slow melting stroke down the hamstring

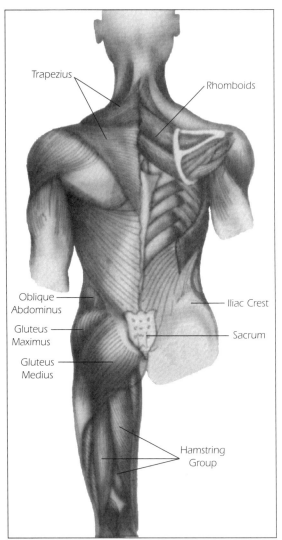

• **Image 36**: *These posterior structures are worked in this session.*

muscle group to a few inches above the knee, where the muscles separate to attach at each side of the knee.

2. Finish with smaller tools sculpting the attachments on the tibia and fibula.

3. If you prefer, work from the knee toward the ischial tuberosity.

Precautions:

1. Remember to avoid deep pressure on

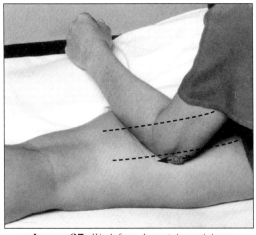

• **Image 37**: *Work from hamstring origin or insertion, according to your preference.*

varicose veins, and redirect sculpting to move in a distal to proximal direction. Eliminate sculpting in this area entirely if severe bulging, ropy varicose veins are present.

2. Avoid direct pressure in the popliteal area of the posterior knee.

<u>*The following procedures are to be done with the client supine*</u>.

5. Lengthening of the quadriceps group myofascia (rectus femoris, vastus lateralis, vastus medialis, vastus intermedius) **(Image 39)**
<u>Intentions and imagery</u>:

1. To elongate the quadriceps group and its investing fascia

2. To release the anterior superior iliac spine (ASIS) from any posterior displacement

3. To connect the torso and legs

<u>Procedures</u>:

1. Begin compressing the origin of the rectus femoris just below the ASIS. Follow any elongating release of the myofascia down toward the knee, or make a series of compressions to just proximal of the patella.

2. Repeat on the vastus medialsis and lateralis.

3. Use a smaller tool to sculpt the attachments of the quadriceps at each side of the patella.

4. Similarly sculpt the other leg.

5. If you prefer, work from the knee toward the pelvis.

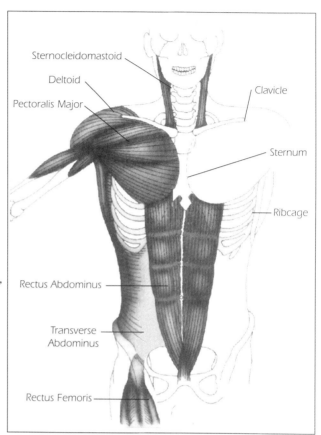

Labels: Sternocleidomastoid, Deltoid, Pectoralis Major, Clavicle, Sternum, Ribcage, Rectus Abdominus, Transverse Abdominus, Rectus Femoris

• **Image 38**: *This session finishes with sculpting anterior structures.*

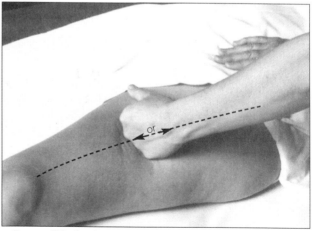

• **Image 39**: *Quadricep muscles also may be sculpted toward the knee or toward the pelvis, as you prefer.*

Precautions: Remember to avoid deep pressure on varicose veins, and redirect sculpting to move in a distal to proximal direction. Eliminate sculpting in this area entirely if severe, bulging, ropy varicose veins are present.

6. Abdominals release (Image 40)

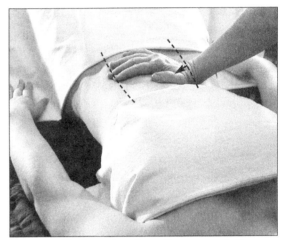

Intention and imagery: To reduce tension in the rectus, oblique, and transverse abdominus muscles and shortening of their interwoven fascia.

Procedure:

1. Use the heel of the hand to compress gently into the abdominal muscles, especially along each edge of the rectus. Make a series of compressions to release the entire abdomen.

2. Compress from near the xyphoid process of the sternum along the inferior edge of the rib cage, releasing the abdominals, especially the rectus and oblique abdominals.

• **Image 40**: *Use only soft, gentle pressure in the abdomen.*

3. Similarly sculpt the other side of the rib cage.

Precautions:

1. Melt slowly to avoid painful pressure on abdominal organs.

2. Do not use this procedure on pregnant or menstruating women, nor with any client experiencing undiagnosed abdominal pain.

3. Avoid painful pressure on the floating eleventh rib by ending the rib cage compressions at the end of the costal cartilages.

7. Anterior flat of the ilium (Image 41)

Intentions and imagery:

1. Skeletal awareness of the pelvis and iliopsoas myofascia

2. Deep release and receptivity into the abdominal muscles

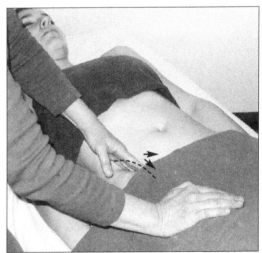

• **Image 41**: *Be sure to wait for yield in the abdominals to avoid forcing into the iliopsoas.*

Procedure:

1. Begin near the anterior superior iliac spine, compressing medial and toward the pubic ramus. Melt slowly and gently into the abdominals then the iliacus, proceeding as the myofascia yields as if "skiing" down the slope of the bowl of the ilium.

2. If release allows you deep enough to contact the psoas muscle, continue in an inferior direction releasing any stringiness, bunching, or tenderness in the psoas.

3. Similarly sculpt the other side.

4. This procedure may be done with the client lying on his side.

Precautions:

1. By entering at the ASIS, keeping the palmar side of your fingers against the flat of the ilium, and reducing pressure if painful, you will avoid any pointed or excessive pressure on abdominal organs.

2. Be especially sensitive to wait for the client's release and to avoid working beyond the client's experience of the "pleasure/pain borderline".

3. Do not apply direct pressure in an inferior direction on the inguinal ligament, as it may be weakened, thereby encouraging herniation.

4. Do not use this procedure on pregnant or menstruating women, nor with any client experiencing undiagnosed abdominal pain.

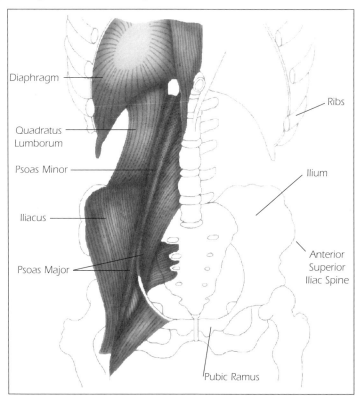

• **Image 42**: *Several intrinsic muscles are involved in this session.*

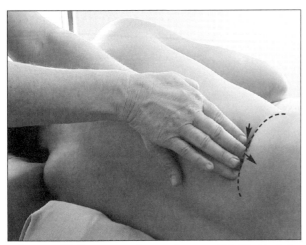

• **Image 43**: *You may prefer your forearm, if it fits, to your fingertips for the quadratus lumborum.*

8. Quadratus lumborum stretch
(Image 43)
<u>Intention and imagery</u>:

1. Release of the quadratus, imagining more space between the ribs and iliac crest and lengthening of the back.

<u>Procedure</u>:

1. Use the forearm or fingertips to compress in a medial and inferior direction on the quadratus.

2. This procedure should be done with client lying on his side.

<u>Hints</u>: The space between the ribs and the pelvis will be smaller on most males than on females due to a difference in the shape of the pelvis. Also, some clients are more shortwaisted than others. If your forearm is too wide or the belly of the muscle cannot be located, work using your fingertips at the origin and insertion.

Strokes to Emphasize for Individual Imbalances
Lumbar lordosis

The excessive lumbar curvature of lordosis is most effectively reduced by sculpting the posterior fascia, the erector spinae, the quadriceps group, and the muscles attaching at the sacrum, the iliac crest, and the anterior surface of the ilium.

When your client's alignment reveals a flattening of the lumbar curve, emphasize sculpting the gluteals and the hamstring group. To change the alignment of the pelvis sufficiently to reduce muscle strain and spasm, encourage iliopsoas toning and stretching.

Other pelvic and spinal imbalances

You will need to relax the quadratus lumborum on the higher side to effect change in uneven iliac crest heights. To release scoliosis, sculpt thoroughly and in detail on the erector spinae, especially on the sides inside the S-curve. The quadratus lumborum also will benefit from careful sculpting.[5]

Supportive Exercises and Stretching
Getting comfortable when in pain

If your client is barely able to move without excruciating lumbar pain, then simply finding a comfortable position in which to rest will be of prime importance. Sidelying in a gentle fetal position can be a neutral, more comfortable resting position. The client should lie on the table, or at home on a bed or sofa, with his knees slightly forward and bent, chin slightly

toward his chest. He may
need pillows under his
head, upper torso,
waistline and/or knees,
and can make other small
adjustments to keep the
entire length of his spine
parallel to the lying
surface. While lying in this
position, breathing should
be conscious, slow, and
deep, but not so deep as
to hurt the back. In this

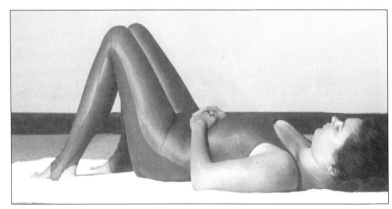

• **Image 44**: *This resting position encourages lumbar elongation and relaxed breathing.*

way, he uses his breath to initiate gentle movement and stretch in the muscles. He can
further stretch his back by delicately and gradually bringing his knees to his chest and/or the
chin to the chest.

Another resting position that can relieve pain, stretch muscles, and relax the client is the
following: The client should lie on his back on a firm surface, knees raised, feet flat on the
table or bed about 12 inches apart. The lower back should be flat, supported by the surface.
The hands rest lightly on the lower abdomen, just below the navel. Deep, diaphragmatic
breathing raises the hands on the belly with each inhale and lowers them with each exhale,
like the movement of waves on the ocean. Breaths should be gentle enough to not raise the
lower back from the bed. The chest should also move gently. **(Image 44)**

Maggie's Back Book: Healing the Hurt in Your Lower Back[6] further elaborates on these
positions, as well as exercise and lifestyle changes. Study of this book and using it with low-
back pain clients is highly recommended.

Muscle strengthening and stretching

Pelvic alignment is primarily created by balance in the functions of antagonist muscles:
the iliopsoas, abdominals, erector spinae, quadriceps, and hamstring groups. Curl-ups,
accomplished while keeping the knees raised, the low back flat on the floor, and by only lifting
the upper body off the floor to approximately scapula level, can usually safely tone the
abdominals. Sit-backs (from seated position with the knees bent, feet on floor, leaning back as
far as needed to engage the abdominals) done to each side, as well as straight backward, are
an even gentler abdominal strengthener.[7]

Practicing pelvic tilting, in lying, standing, and on all-fours positions, uses the iliopsoas for
pelvic positioning on the frontal plane and strengthens this muscle unit. In the supine position
with knees up as described above, the pelvic tilt can most easily be practiced, because the
shoulders and hips are stabilized and gravity assists the posterior tilting of the pelvic crest.
The client should roll his pelvis back gently at the crests, as his lower back flattens down on

the lying surface. An image of tucking a tail between the legs suggests this movement, as does imagining that the sacrum is a flat ice cream scoop shaving off a very thin layer of ice cream from the surface as it moves. Done subtly as described above, this type of pelvic tilt reeducates the movement patterns to effectively use the iliopsoas for balanced pelvic alignment. If the abdominals are tightened and the tilt exaggerated, then abdominals and psoas both are toned by this exercise.

Knee-to-chest stretches elongate lumbar and the hamstring myofascia. Modifying this stretch by bringing the knee across the midline, stretches the medial hip rotators, part of the quadratus lumborum, and the latissimus dorsi. A sink, or something sturdily attached to a wall, can be an anchoring spot for a full back and buttocks stretch. While grasping the sink firmly at about arms' length, the knees are bent, head and bottom are tucked under. With small, careful side-to-side movements, the hips are leaned backward and stretched toward the opposite wall. The lower back is always rounded and the pelvis tucked under as the stretch is deepened with more bend in the knees, greater traction and slow, conscious, full breathing. Stretches appropriate for clients with low-back discomfort are elaborated in *Stretching*,[8] *Maggie's Back Book*, and in *Relaxercise*.[9]

An easy stretch for the quadriceps group happens when grasping the ankle and bringing it to near the buttock while standing. Further stretch in this position can release the ilopsoas. Remind clients to not bounce during stretches, and to use slow, deliberate, full breathing while stretching for 30-45 seconds. Another option is to actively stretch the muscle after 2-5 seconds of muscle use against resistence.

Double leg raises from a prone position and conventional sit-ups primarily strengthen the hip flexors rather than the abdominals, and often produce a strain on the lower back. These exercises should be avoided.

Healthy backs can benefit from more strenuous exercise and stretching. Safe leg lowering and scissoring require strong abdominals to maintain the lower back flat against the floor. These are considerably more strenuous exercises, as are some of the very effective yoga stretches and exercises such as the Shoulder-stand, Plow, Salute to the Sun, and Udiyama. Movements that twist, rotate, flex, and extend the spine (such as the Ax and lateral stretch in Arica Psychocalisthenics[sm] [10] increase spinal mobility and torso muscle strength.

Situations to Avoid and Everyday Considerations

Clients with low-back pain may need discussion about and evaluation of their everyday activities, environments, and habits to eliminate possible causes and factors contributing to their pain. They should avoid high heels, girdles, leaning forward from the waist, lifting without squatting, toe touching and double leg raising exercise, rigid and cross-legged sitting positions, carrying heavy loads, and being overweight. Clients also may need advice in choice of beds, chairs, and how to accomplish routine tasks such as brushing teeth and taking a bath without further pain and injury. (See *Maggie's Back Book* and *Relaxercise*.)

Body/Mind Connections

Most somatic psychologies suggest that fear—of life, vitality, and sexuality—is held in tightened muscles of the pelvic area, especially the gluteals, the intrinsic pelvic muscles, and the pelvic floor. Nerves from the lumbar spine activate the sexual and eliminative functions, as well as the legs and feet. Rigidity and imbalance in this area can block the pelvis from free movement, thereby inhibiting fluid walking, dancing, and sexual expression.

Since lumbar alignment is a function of balance between the anterior and posterior musculature, abdominal correlations also need to be considered. Generally, the abdomen is associated with issues of nourishment and assimilation of emotions, as well as food. Thus, lumbar tension might suggest exploring the client's unexpressed emotions concerning nurturance and sexuality.[11] (See Chapter Four, pp. 48-56 for further elaboration.)

Sources Cited

[1] *Postgraduate Medicine Journal*, 1981.

[2] Godfrey, C.M., P.P. Morgan, and J. Schatzker. "A randomized trial of manipulation for low-back pain in a medical setting." *Spine*, 1984:9, pp.301-304.

[3] Field, Tiffany, Iris Burman, et.al. *International Journal of Neuroscience*, 106: 2001, pp.131-145.

[4] Cherkin DC, D. Eisenberg, K.J. Sherman, W. Barlow, T.J. Kaptchuk, J. Street, R.A. Deyo. "Randomized trial comparing traditional Chinese medical acupuncture, therapeutic massage, and self-care education for chronic low back pain." *Archives of Internal Medicine*, 2001:161, pp.1081-1088.

[5] For another insightful look at myofascial lengthening in the low back area see Alexander, Doug. "Lengthening Stereotypes," *Massage Therapy Journal*, Summer, 1999: Vol. 38, 2, pp.40-54.

[6] Leavin, Maggie. *Maggie's Back Book: Healing the Hurt in Your Lower Back*. Boston, MA: Houghton Mifflin Company, 1976.

[7] For other awareness and releasing exercises specifically for the psoas muscle, see Koch, Liz. *The Psoas Book* (Second Edition), Felton, CA: Guinea Pig Publications, 1997.

[8] Anderson, Bob. *Stretching*. Bolinas, CA: Shelter Publications, Inc., 1980.

[9] Zemach-Bersin, David, Kaethe Zemach-Bersin, and Mark Reese. *Relaxercise*. New York, NY: HarperCollins Publishers, 1990.

[10] Ichazo, Oscar. *Psychocalisthenics*. New York, NY: Simon and Schuster, 1976.

[11] Dychtwald, Kenneth. *Body/Mind*. New York, NY: Jove Publications, Inc., 1977, especially Chapter 5.

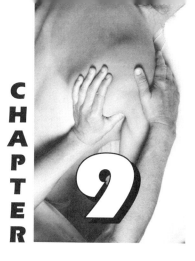

CHAPTER

2

Deep Tissue Sculpting Session for the Neck and Shoulders

The universality of neck and shoulder tension in Western cultures is, in part, the reflection of sedentary lifestyles and of centuries-old religious, philosophical, and scientific beliefs fostering a separation between mind/emotions and body. Verbal expression also flows or is blocked in the throat and neck. The neck is a major thoroughfare in transporting nourishment and oxygen to the brain, air to the lungs, and food to the digestive organs. Since Western society is so head-dominated, it is no wonder that neck injury, degenerative conditions, chronic headaches, vision and hearing deficiencies, sinus congestion, TMJ, and other common complaints are produced or exacerbated by chronic neck and shoulder tension.

Guiding Imagery for the Session:
Lengthen the Neck; Center the Head; Drop the Shoulders

Structural evaluation of clients who present neck and shoulder discomfort will usually reveal anterior or posterior displacement of the head on the atlas vertebra, and often displacement of the entire cervical spine. Flattening of the cervical curvature, or lordosis, in this area of the spine also is common as gravity relentlessly presses down, and tensions in the flexors or extensors of the neck exert their pull. Elevation of the shoulders is common, since the trapezius and levator scapula are almost universally in chronic contracture. Thus, the image or intention to be held as your guiding thought while working will be to lengthen the neck, center the head, and drop the shoulders. Your client also might be engaged in imagining these changes as you work together.

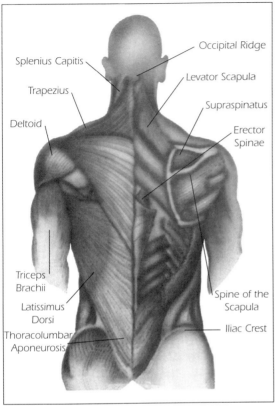

Splenius Capitis
Trapezius
Deltoid
Triceps Brachii
Latissimus Dorsi
Thoracolumbar Aponeurosis

Occipital Ridge
Levator Scapula
Supraspinatus
Erector Spinae
Spine of the Scapula
Iliac Crest

• **Image 45**: *Several layers of posterior structures are involved in this session.*

The procedures explained below are all designed to facilitate tension reduction in the neck and shoulders. Observation and evaluation of the individual client should guide you in determining which of these are appropriate and most effective for that client; some might be omitted, and others might be emphasized.

The procedures listed are only deep tissue sculpting procedures. Include initial contact, integrative and transitional procedures, and closure interactions when working with your client. There are other types of soft tissue therapies that you might integrate into these procedures or blend together to further enhance their effect. Several of these techniques also may be effective as part of a primarily circulatory or passive movement massage session, for example. Create and integrate sculpting as part of an eclectic bodywork approach to the individuals with whom you work. (See Chapter Eleven, pp. 117-136.)

The following procedures are to be done with the client in the supine position. Use elbow, forearm, fist, knuckle, or finger, depending on your client's and your relative sizes and the depth of structure to be sculpted. Dashed lines on photos represent areas to sculpt; solid arrows denote vector of pressure to apply.

1. Occipital ridge (Image 46)

Intention and imagery: To release tension in fascial and muscle attachments at the occipital ridge and mastoid processes, especially trapezius, sternocleidomastoid, splenius capitis, and suboccipitals; more length in the back of the neck and more space in the spine.

Procedure: Compress into muscle attachments at the occipital ridge, using the fingertips of both hands. Begin at the midpoint of the ridge, and continue laterally to the mastoid process with a series of compressions.

Precautions:

1. Avoid hair pulling and ear mashing.

2. Do not yank or over-stretch the spine with traction. Use a very gradual shifting of your weight back away from the table.

Hints:

1. Do not lift the head from the table. Your arms will remain more relaxed without the weight of the head. Position your hands at the side of the head either posterior of or cupping the ears, and reach with your fingertips to the occipital ridge.

2. Use gentle, moderate traction on the spine to increase pressure as tissue softens and lengthens.

3. One side then the other may be worked rather than sculpting with both hands simultaneously.

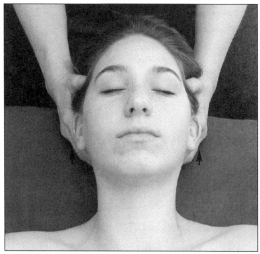

• **Image 46**: *Position your hands for occipital ridge sculpting by encircling the ears.*

For the rest of the session you may choose to do one side and then the other for each procedure. Or do all seven of them in sequence on one side, then repeat the sequence on the other side before turning the client over for the final back procedure.

2. Upper trapezius myofascia (Image 47)

(A supine version of the same procedure as in session for release of the back.)

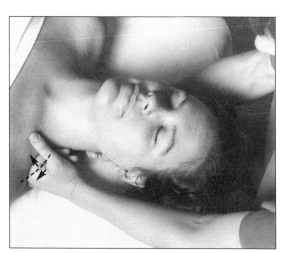

Intention and imagery: To elongate the upper trapezius fibers, allowing the shoulders to drop and broaden.

Procedure: Compress and/or stroke the trapezius from near the neck to the acromioclavicular joint.

Precautions: Avoid excess pressure on the brachial plexus and carotid artery by working posterior of these structures.

Hints:

1. Do not use so deep a compression as to bump over the deeper lying muscles.

2. This stroke may be done with the client prone or on her side.

• **Image 47**: *Note that upper trapezius sculpting avoids excess direct pressure on vulnerable vascular and neural structures.*

3. Superior spine of the scapula attachments (Image 48)

(A supine version of the same procedure as in session for release of the back.)

<u>Intention and imagery</u>: To increase skeletal awareness of the scapula, and to relax the trapezius attachments and supraspinatus muscle on the spine of the scapula, allowing the shoulders to drop and broaden.

<u>Procedure</u>: Compress and/or stroke along the superior edge of the spine of the scapula, moving laterally out to

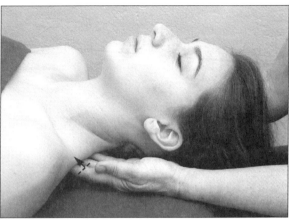

• **Image 48**: *The superior spine of the scapula tapers at its lateral end, requiring smaller tools there.*

the acromioclavicular joint. Change tools as necessary to fit the gradually narrowing space.

4. Levator scapulae attachment (Image 49)

<u>Intention and imagery</u>: To clear the levator scapulae attachment on the scapula, allowing the shoulders to drop and broaden.

<u>Procedure</u>:

1. Locate the superior angle of the scapula, and compress and release the levator insertion and any accompanying bunched fascia with your fingertips.

2. For an anterior entry to this muscle, use your thumb to release the mid-portion of the levator by compressing on the shoulder just anterior to the trapezius and toward the levator insertion.

<u>Precautions</u>: Avoid excess pressure on the brachial plexus and carotid artery by working posterior of these structures and directing pressure posterior. Ask for client feedback.

<u>Hints</u>:

1. Melt slowly and carefully in this especially tight muscle.

2. Though you may not reach the insertion with the anterior entry, direct your pressure toward the superior angle of the scapula. You may want to keep your fingertips on this area to help your aim, but this is not

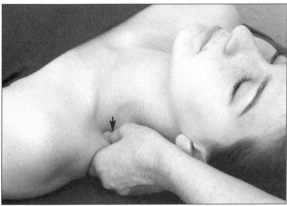

• **Image 49**: *Precise placement and direction is necessary when approaching the levator scapula from the anterior.*

to be a squeezing of the trapezius and levator between the thumbs and fingertips.

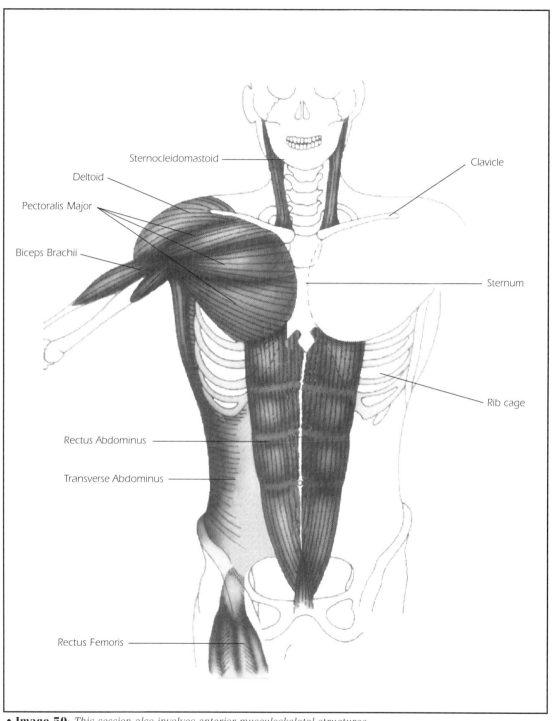

Sternocleidomastoid

Clavicle

Deltoid

Pectoralis Major

Biceps Brachii

Sternum

Rib cage

Rectus Abdominus

Transverse Abdominus

Rectus Femoris

• **Image 50**: *This session also involves anterior musculoskeletal structures.*

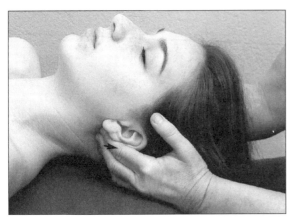

• **Image 51**: *While one hand sculpts the SCM insertion, the other helps balance and support the head.*

5. Sternocleidomastoid

(SCM)attachments **(Image 51)**

<u>Intention and imagery</u>: To release tension in the SCM, allowing for more balanced placement of the head on the atlas vertebra and more horizontal alignment of the shoulders.

<u>Procedure</u>: Compress with the thumbs or fingertips at the insertion at the mastoid process and the origin on the medial clavicle.

<u>Precautions</u>:

1. Do not work both sides of the neck together since deeper pressure on both may unnecessarily restrict blood flow to the brain.

2. With clients that are obese, formerly obese, or clients 60 years of age or older, take care to not stroke down the SCM, since any arterial plaque might be loosened.

3. Direct your stroke in an inferior direction rather than medial, as pressure on the esophagus may trigger a cough reflex.

4. Ask for feedback regarding any numbness, pain, or electrical sensations that might be felt down the arm signaling brachial plexus compression. Change direction of pressure if necessary to avoid pressure on the brachial plexus.

6. Defining the clavicle (Image 52)

<u>Intention and imagery</u>: To increase skeletal awareness of the clavicle and to relax attaching muscles and fascia; to encourage the clavicles to drop to a more horizontal and level position.

<u>Procedure</u>: Compress with the fingertips along the superior edge of the clavicle, releasing tension in the attaching muscles. Move from near the sternal notch to the acromioclavicular joint.

<u>Precautions</u>:

1. Ask for feedback regarding any numbness, pain, or electrical sensations that might be felt down the arm signaling brachial plexus compression. Change direction of pressure if necessary to avoid

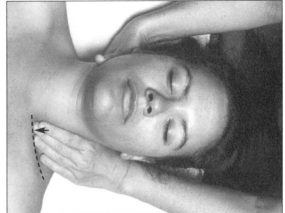

• **Image 52**: *Clavicle sculpting must also be precisely and sensitively performed to avoid the vulnerable vascular and neural structures.*

pressure on the brachial plexus. Ask for client feedback.

2. Continue compressions into the "V" formed by the articulation of the clavicle and scapula, taking care to avoid strain to the ligamental structure of this joint.

7. Pectoralis major myofascia (Image 53)

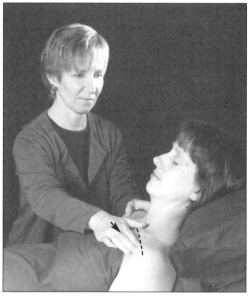

Intention and imagery: To elongate the pectoralis major, opening the chest and pectoral girdle.

Procedure: Compress and/or stroke from the attachments on the sternum and clavicle, following the anterior fascia and the pectoralis major to its insertion on the humerus.

Hints:

1. On females, compress only the origins at the sternum and costal cartilage and the humeral insertion to avoid compressing breast tissue, except the most superior fibers which may be stroked or compressed as on males.

2. If body hair is pulled uncomfortably, either do not stroke the muscle or use a slight amount of oil on the hair.

• **Image 53**: *For best body usage, sculpt the pectoralis major on the opposite side from where you are standing.*

8. Opening down the arm (Image 54)

Intention and imagery: To release the flexor and extensor myofascia of the arm, and thereby elongate the arm and open a channel of energy from the heart area down the arms and out the hands.

Procedure:

1. Compress and/or stroke from the deltoids down the biceps brachii and hand flexors.

2. Turn the arm to sculpt from the deltoids down the triceps and hand extensors.

Precautions: Lighten pressure over the elbow and wrist to avoid uncomfortable pressures and positions in these joints.

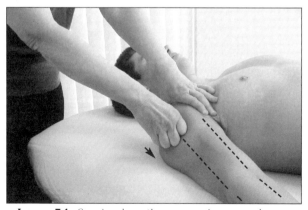

• **Image 54**: *Opening down the arm requires several repositionings of the client's arm and your stance.*

The following procedure is to be done in the prone or sidelying position.

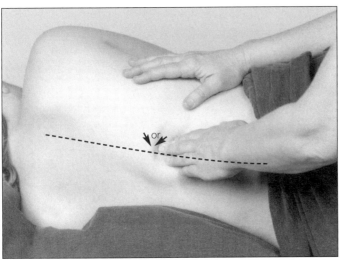

• **Image 55**: _Lengthening the back may be performed in the sidelying position, as can many of the techniques in all three sessions in Chapters Seven, Eight, and Nine._

9. Lengthening the back

(Image 55) (Same procedure as in sessions for release of the back and the lower back).

<u>Intention and imagery</u>: To elongate and relax the muscles and fascia attaching to and paralleling the spine, primarily the posterior fascia, trapezius, thorocolumbar aponeurosis, rhomboids, and erector spinae.

<u>Procedure</u>:

1. From a position in front of the client's head, begin stroking/compressing along the tissues lateral to the spine.

2. Continue from near the C-7 area to the base of the sacrum, changing tools as muscles narrow above and over the sacrum.

<u>Precautions</u>:

1. Do not stroke directly over spinous processes, but instead apply pressure lateral of them.

2. In the lumbar area, be sure to direct pressure more toward the sacrum than in an anterior direction to avoid excessively curving the lower back.

3. If lumbar lordosis is extreme, support the area with a folded towel or a small pillow beneath the abdomen, or do this and all other prone procedures with the client in a sidelying position.

<u>Hints</u>:

1. You may work both simultaneously, or left then right sides of the back.

2. As with all sculpting, do not force an unbroken stroke if the tissue is not elongating. A series of compressions is equally as effective, and a combination of stroking and compressions will more likely be the pattern of release.

3. Change tools as needed to accommodate body position and to avoid excessive leaning over the table.

Techniques to Emphasize for Each Misalignment

Address elevation of the shoulders by emphasizing the release of the upper fibers of the trapezius, trapezius attachments, and the more intrinsic levator scapulae. Posterior displacement of the head on the atlas requires release of the sternocleidomastoid, while the occipital ridge, trapezius, and erector spinae must elongate and relax to relieve anterior displacement. If the head is chronically rotated to one side, then the trapezius on the side toward which rotation occurs and the SCM on the opposite side will need the most emphasis. Relaxation of the SCM, and the trapezius on the side to which the head is tilted, will help to correct a lateral tilt of the head on the atlas. If the chin is elevated, thoroughly sculpt the occipital ridge and upper trapezius.

Supportive Exercises and Stretching

The supine position recommended for low-back tension also is useful as a resting position for discomfort in the neck. **(Image 44, p.97)** Attention should be focused on allowing the posterior neck to be supported by the floor or table. In acute neck spasm, clients will need to be especially careful to roll to their side and push with the arms to a seated position, rather than doing a sit-up when leaving this position.

Tai chi chuan offers an image of spinal alignment that encourages a balanced head position on the axis. A weight is imagined as attaching to the coccyx. Its weight pulls earthward, lengthening the spine. A hook is simultaneously imagined as attaching to the crown of the head and continuing up toward the sky. This skyhook extends the spine, while it also aligns the head by tending to slightly tuck the chin. The skyhook image affords a lengthening of the spine from the relentless downward press felt from gravity, without the excessive tightening of the neck that the "head back, chest up, stomach in" military posture often creates. This complementary earthward and skyward extension of the spine creates lift and grounding in the individual's structure and energy field.

The tense/release exercise of holding the shoulders as high toward the ears as possible for 5-10 seconds then releasing downward can help relax tight shoulders. Resisting this motion by holding the shoulder down with the opposite arm also lengthens trapezius, levator scapula, and supraspinatus muscles. Use similar exercises on other tight muscles to further their relaxation. Smoothly rolling the pectoral girdle through forward rotation, elevation, retraction, and depression, then repeating forward and elevation movements during inhalation, with a sharp exhalation as the shoulders are finally dropped again, also can be effective. This type of shoulder roll and the head series from Arica Psychocalisthenics[1] should be done gently and without pain, only within a comfortable range of movement. Healthier necks, shoulders, and upper backs can retain flexibility with Shoulderstand, Plow, and other yoga postures.

Stretching the neck in all directions of movement must be accomplished with attention to breathing fully and nonstressfully, as gentle elongation is encouraged in 30-45 second stretches. Areas of pain and limitation of movement must be respected to avoid further acute spasm. *Stretching*[2] and *Relaxercise*[3] detail various positions for stretching specific areas of the neck and shoulders.

Situations to Avoid and Everyday Considerations

Many people continually strain their neck during passive, relaxing activities such as sleeping, reading, and television viewing. Extreme positions of flexion and extension of the neck and tilts of the head should be avoided by using pillows, beds, and chairs that support the cervical spine and head in balanced alignment. Persons in seated occupations especially secretaries, computer workers, and receptionists may need to have their work stations evaluated so that chair, desk, and equipment height, position, and usage will not contribute to neck and shoulder strain.

Body/Mind Connection

Most somatic psychologies expect shoulder tension to be related to fears of responsibility and a feeling of burden. Elevation of the shoulders is frequently found to be reflective of chronic fear. When thoughts, beliefs, and intellectual considerations control one's life with little regard for the emotions or physical needs, then it is almost impossible to be wholly present in one's life. Neck and shoulder tension blocks messages from the torso and the lower body, thereby fostering a "head" orientation to living. Additionally, when emotionally overwhelmed, expression is often blocked by tension in the neck and throat. (See Chapter Four, pp. 48-56 for further elaboration.) Again, regardless of what the theory states, the individual's emotional experience is most relevant.

Sources Cited

[1] Ichazo, Oscar. *Psychocalisthenics.* New York, NY: Simon and Schuster, 1976.

[2] Anderson, Bob. *Stretching.* Bolinas, CA: Shelter Publications, Inc., 1980.

[3] Zemach-Bersin, David, Kaethe Zemach-Bersin, and Mark Reese. *Relaxercise.* New York: NY, HarperCollins Publishers, 1990.

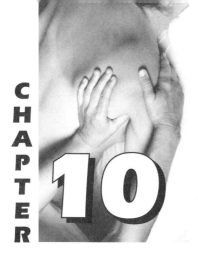

10 Full Body Sculpting and Applications to Other Body Areas

Full Body Sculpting Session

Many practitioners will find that a single session of deep tissue sculpting is all that a particular individual will schedule. Some clients also have no specific area of pain, but report a generalized sensation of tension all over the body. These and other situations may call for sculpting the full body rather than the specialized areas taught in the preceding chapters.

A full body sculpting session can take as long as two hours to complete; however, most practitioners will be able to sensitively and effectively work the key areas in a one-hour session. Because most of these procedures were elaborated in the preceding chapters, only brief descriptions are listed here.

The procedures listed below lead the practitioner from the head to the feet, sculpting first the anterior of the body then the posterior. However, it might be more appropriate to reverse this order with some clients or to arrange in other formats.

Procedures with the client in the supine position

1. Initial Contact: Center yourself and establish receptive, respectful contact with your client.
2. Compress and release the muscle and fascial attachments at the occipital ridge of the skull. (See Chapter Nine, pp. 102-103 for detail.)
3. Sculpt and relax the upper trapezius from near the neck to the acromioclavicular joint. (See Chapter Nine, p. 103 for detail.)
4. Sculpt the forehead, temples, and cheekbones with gentle compressions, moving lateral from the midline of the face and from the hairline to the mouth.
5. Compress down the arms from shoulder to hands on either the inside or outside of the arm. (See Chapter Nine, p. 107 for details.)
6. Sculpt between the metacarpals. (Repeat steps 5 and 6 on the other arm.)

7. Compress gently along the lateral edges of the rectus abdominus to relax the abdominals. (See Chapter Eight, p. 94 for details.)
8. Sculpt and relax the quadriceps from origin to insertion above the knee. (See Chapter Eight, pp. 93-94 for details.)
9. Sculpt and release the attachments on the anterior of the the tibia, moving proximal to distal.
10. Sculpt between the metatarsals. (Repeat steps 8-10 on the other leg.)

Procedures with the client in the prone position

11. Compress under and release the attachments along the vertebral border of the scapula. (See Chapter Seven, p. 81 for details.)
12. Lengthen the back by sculpting and elongating the erector spinae and associated fascia from the shoulders to the sacrum. (See Chapter Seven, p. 82 for details.)
13. Compress and/or stroke the gluteus maximus from origin toward the insertion into the iliotibial tract, elongating and melting the muscle and fascia. (See Chapter Seven, p. 84 for details.)
14. Lengthen the hamstring group from ischial tuberosities to just above the knee. (See Chapter Eight, pp. 92-93 for details.)
15. Sculpt and release the gastrocnemius from origin to insertion. (Repeat steps 13, 14, and 15 on the other leg.)
16. Complete the session with gentle, soothing contact on the soles of both feet.

Using Basic Principles for Applications with Other Body Areas

Over 26 years of clinical experience indicate that 50% or more of clients use massage therapy for tension relief in the neck and upper back. Approximately 30% of massage therapy clients seek relief from low back pain and disability. The remaining 20% of a therapeutic practice typically addresses leg, arm, and facial tension. This book has focused on specific effective techniques for working with these areas of typical tension.

The basic bodywork and sculpting principles detailed in Chapter Two can guide you to appropriate work in any area of the body. The following specific example will illustrate how to apply those principles to sculpt in areas other than those specified in preceding chapters.

Sharon is a real estate agent who cannot resist buying "fixer-upper" properties and transforming them. Masonry projects, from entry ways to garden walls and chimneys, are especially attractive to her. Her hands and forearms, however, began protesting these labors of love. Scraping, chiseling, and forming the mortar resulted in muscle tension and ligament sprain, particularly in her forearms and the opponens pollicis muscle. How could you utilize sculpting to relieve her arms and hands?

Technique follows perception which is a function of love.

First observe the presenting body part, in this case the hand and forearm, the whole individual, and the relevant history of the client with respect, intuition, acuity, and love. Let your observations lead you to appropriate therapeutic action. In this case, the most effective work would likely include deep tissue sculpting, supplemented by circulatory, trigger point and cross-fiber techniques to relieve chronic tension, waste product buildup, referred pain, and adhesion in the connective tissue. Attend to any emotional tensions that may surface.

What one imagines or visualizes is what will be touched or created.

Sculpting the hand necessitates precisely visualizing the wrist joint, fingers, fascia, and fibers of the specific muscles being worked, such as the opponens pollicis. See that muscle as perfectly aligned and elongated as in an anatomy text, and let that image guide you toward that result.

The balance of receptive and active energies is the process of bodywork.

Encourage your client to participate in elongating the opponens pollicis through deep abdominal breathing, visualizing that effect, and movement. Use strength from your legs to softly melt layer by layer into the skin, superficial fascia, and finally the muscle and myofascia.

Pressure is usually applied paralleling muscle fibers and/or following the bone structure.

Sculpt the fibers of the opponens pollicis from near the first metacarpal/phalangeal joint, following as they parallel the metacarpal bone.

Strokes and compressions are done with increasing pressure only to a level of balance between release and resistance.

Use a perceived pain indicator scale of either numbers or colors, or solicit other feedback to maintain an intensity level of pleasure/pain as the opponens pollicis relaxes.

The release of the tissue guides the speed, direction, and depth of all techniques.

Go further along or deeper in only when sinking and melting to deeper levels occurs. Avoid pushing and forcing.

Using similar steps as in the above example, any area of chronic tension and myofascial restriction may be released with deep tissue sculpting.

Tableside Technique Guide

Deep Tissue Sculpting Session for the Neck and Shoulders ▪ Chapter Nine Procedures (pp. 101-108)
Guiding Imagery for Session: Lengthen the Neck; Center the Head; Drop the Shoulders

	PROCEDURE	INTENTION	VECTOR	HINTS AND PRECAUTIONS
1	defining the occipital ridge	more length and space in neck and spine	anterior then cephalic traction	gradual traction
2	upper trapezius myofascia	drop and broaden shoulders	inferior and lateral	avoid excess pressure on brachial plexus, carotid artery
3	superior spine of the scapula attachments	drop and broaden shoulders	inferior and lateral	moderate pressure at acromioclavicular joint
4	levator scapulae attachments	drop and broaden shoulders	#1-caudal #2-posterior and caudal	avoid excess pressure on brachial plexus, carotid artery
5	sternocleidomastoid attachments	center the head and drop the shoulders	on mastoid-medial on clavicle-caudal	work unilaterally on attachments only; caution re: brachial plexus, esophagus
6	defining the clavicle	center the head and drop the shoulders	caudal	caution re: brachial plexus and acromioclavicular joint
7	pectoralis major myofascia	opening the chest and arms	posterior and lateral	avoid compressing breast tissue and brachial plexus
8	opening down the arm	opening the chest and connecting down the arms	distal	watch pressure on wrist and elbow
9	lengthening the back	lengthen the back	caudal or cranial and anterior	avoid excess anterior pressure in lumbar

ASSIMILATING

- Integrating Deep Tissue Sculpting into a Practice

- Customizing Sculpting for Individual Clients

- In Conclusion: Coming Full Circle

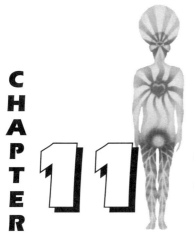

CHAPTER 11

Integrating Deep Tissue Sculpting into a Practice

In the preceding chapters, only sculpting procedures have been used in the sessions presented. For the purpose of understanding and embodying the generalities, as well as the subtleties, of this approach, this exclusivity is appropriate. In practice, however, most practitioners augment their sculpting by using it in conjunction with other body therapy styles. The many essential similarities in massage, soft tissue manipulations, and other somatic therapies allow for effectively integrating different modalities in single sessions or in a series of sessions with an individual client. Often, specific, appropriate techniques from several modalities used together can be the most effective response to the client's presenting concern. For example, sculpting blends exceptionally well with passive movement, and integrates with skin rolling and other forms of deep tissue work. Structural balancing, deep transverse friction, trigger point therapy, and positional release and other osteopathic soft tissue modalities integrate well with sculpting. General guidance for integrating these and other modalities are described later in this chapter.

Sculpting also can enhance other healthcare providers' effectiveness. Interviews with many practitioners throughout the U.S. and Canada have indicated that they are utilizing sculpting compatibly in collaborations with psychotherapists and other mental health professionals, physicians, dentists, chiropractors, and various maternity care providers. These practitioners, as well as physical therapists, nurses, athletic trainers, and exercise and fitness instructors, sometimes learn sculpting to add to their own hands-on skills.

Sculpting is an effective technique for practitioners working in almost any setting from private practices, collaborative and integrative healthcare clinics, spas and resorts, on-site in businesses, and in athletic facilities.

Swedish Massage

Swedish massage involves various kneading (petrissage), rolling, gliding (effleurage), vibration, and percussive movements applied to the skin and underlying soft tissues. These techniques can be used prior to sculpting to increase circulation in the area to be sculpted, to provide preliminary identification of spasmed muscles, and to gradually introduce the client to deeper and slower pressures as transition is made into deep tissue sculpting. Because the circulatory effects of sculpting are probably minimal and mostly quite localized, another option is to follow sculpting with effleurage and kneading to flush the sculpted area, and

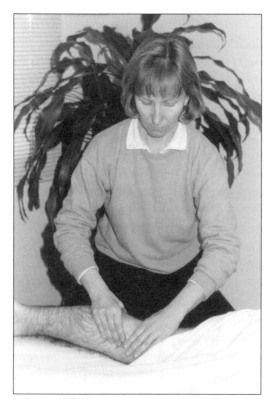

• **Image 56**: *Swedish massage strokes effectively integrate with sculpting.*

to increase circulation that may help remove waste products.[1]

When combining sculpting and Swedish work, reduce lubricant used to the barest amount necessary to create glide during Swedish techniques. This will help prevent sliding on the skin instead of the desired myofascial change sought when sculpting. Another option is to remove oil or lotion before sculpting or only apply after sculpting to finish with Swedish techniques. Petrissage, kneading, and other compression techniques also can be modified to be done without oil. **(Image 56)**

Passive and Active Movement

Passive and active movement methods for balancing the body/mind are especially effective when integrated with sculpting. In passive movements systems, the practitioner lifts, tractions, rocks, and mobilizes the client with no effort from the client. Passive movement systems include psychophysical integration (as developed by Milton Trager),[2] Japanese trepidations, passive joint movements, and sensory repatterning (as developed by James Stewart at the International Professional School of Bodywork).[3]

While sensitively mobilizing the client's joints and creating slow gestures, both you and your client can more precisely identify restricted areas; subsequent sculpting is then more specific. Gentle rocking and undulating movements interrupt the client's proprioceptive "right feeling" that is signaled by habitual patterns, thereby increasing movement possibilities. After sculpting, performing rhythmic passive movements allows the client to explore and experience the resulting elongation and separation in neighboring muscle groups on a kinesthetic level. When you reintroduce functionally efficient movement patterns, you also reeducate motor responses and generate more individualized, freer movement possibilities for the client.[4]

In addition to alternating use of passive movement and sculpting, as described above, you can blend sculpting simultaneously with this type of movement. Typically one hand sensitively melts into a localized

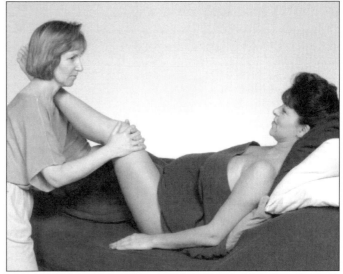

• **Image 57**: *Active muscle use against the practitioner's resistance is one form of movement to integrate with sculpting.*

myofascial restriction. This begins the process of inducing the reflex relaxation response and helps unravel the myofascial components of the restriction. While maintaining consistent sculpting pressure, use your other hand to gently grasp a body part adjacent to the restricted area, initiating small amplitude, slowly paced, undulating gestures of passive movement. These movements tend to create a meditative alertness, a distraction, and a neurological willingness to release habitual structural tendencies. This creates an integrative and, in effect, a neuromuscular response in the client.[5]

In injured tissues, use of blended or alternating sculpting and passive movement helps to maximize tissue repair by increasing local circulation to damaged muscle and connective tissue. As soft tissues heal, platelets, macrophages, and mast cells vigorously restore normal tissue. Fibroblasts lay down collagen.

After the acute injury phase, blended work facilitates the repair along normal fiber direction thus reducing immobility due to accumulated collagen adhesions (scar tissue or fibrosis). Passive movements shift the muscles in their fascial sheaths as fibrotic areas are compressed and softened with sculpting. This combination of subtle movement and persistent pressure gently frees myofascial restrictions and facilitates normal tissue healing.

Passive and active stretching and range of motion exercise can also reinforce and maintain elongation and space after sculpting. Active types of movements involve the client's own contractile muscular action. **(Image 57)** Specific stretches for the sculpted muscle creates a pull on connective tissue, warming it and increasing its thixotrophic response. Range of motion exercises, resisted exercises, and either passive or active movements help both client and practitioner to assess movement potential prior to and following sculpting and other bodywork techniques.[6]

Other Deep Tissue Methodologies

Some Rolfing, Postural Integration, structural balancing or integration, myofascial, and Hellerwork practitioners find deep tissue sculpting compatible with the variation of deep tissue work that they predominately practice. Where sensitive, yet penetrating pressure is called for, sculpting can open the client's receptivity and prepare the tissue for the oftentimes more aggressive techniques of some of these methodologies. Equally as complementary, predominantly sculpting practitioners might include in their intention and technique the basic principles of alignment and movement as elaborated by Rolf or her many followers.[7]

Deep muscular therapy (developed by Ben Benjamin), deep transverse friction (developed by James Cyriax), myofascial release (developed by John Barnes), neuromuscular technique (developed by Leon Chaitow, Paul St. John, Judith DeLany, and others), and trigger point therapy (developed by Janet Travell) integrate well with sculpting techniques. As you slowly sculpt, areas of chronic tension and specific points of tenderness can be identified and precisely located. After melting the area with sculpting, facilitate further breakdown of adhesion in these areas with transverse friction and other techniques. Ligaments involved can be similarly treated.

When your sculpting uncovers trigger points, hypersensitive areas that usually refer pain, maintain your pressure precisely on the trigger point. Ask your client to report the gradual desensitization and relief of pain that usually occurs. Maintain your ischemic compression of the point for 7-20 seconds after it is at least 75% less painful, and then proceed with your sculpting. Very active trigger points are often most permanently extinguished with additional passive stretching of the involved tissue with or without the use of vaso-coolant sprays.

Skin Rolling

Sometimes tension in the skin and superficial fascia must be released in order to work into the deep fascia and musculature. These areas of reduced elasticity and adherence to the underlying tissues are common with chronic pain syndromes, recurrent headaches, and some organic dysfunctions.[8] Psychological tension frequently alters the skin motility and flexibility as well.[9]

Begin skin rolling by lifting the tight skin into a welt between both thumbs and the index and middle fingers. Move this roll of skin and underlying fascia along to loosen restricted and bound areas. Allow the fingers to feed tissue towards the thumbs as they maintain a slow, gentle, constant pressure, creating a rolling movement. Sometimes holding in particularly glued spots for 30 seconds or more can relax areas of superficial fascial restriction. Be sure to moderate pressure and speed of rolling so that the client's perceived pain level doesn't exceed pleasure-on-the-borderline-of-pain. Create other variations by changing the angle of stretch and pull, the direction of rolling, and the depth of tissue grasped.

Roll the entire body, or work with regional areas of stuck, tight skin. Follow rolling with the sculpting techniques of this manual into the deeper tissues.

Oriental Body Therapies

Practitioners who are familiar with meridian-based body therapies often find that while slowly sculpting, meridian points may be areas of tension and tenderness. Precise and direct pressure as well as the gradual, deep release of sculpting are often required in these areas. Practitioners familiar with both Eastern and Western methodologies often use a sculpting-like pressure following various meridians as a method of opening the flow along these energy pathways.

Emotional Processing Methodologies

As detailed in Chapter Four, sculpting and somato-emotional integration are naturally compatible methodologies. Those suggestions for facilitating emotional responses aroused during sculpting work provide adequate guidelines and strategies. For those practitioners motivated to more actively incorporate feeling, sensation, and memory processing, more comprehensive training in this type of work should be pursued. Recommended programs are available through the integrative somatics curriculum of the International

Professional School of Bodywork (including courses with the author, Edward Maupin, Diana Panara, and James Stewart),[10] Ilana Rubenfeld's Rubenfeld Synergy Center,[11] Ron Kurtz's Hakomi Institute,[12] and Peter Levine's Foundation for Human Enrichment.[13] There also are elements of this type of work in the Upledger somatoemotional release trainings[14] and John Barnes' myofascial unwinding.[15]

Many forms of therapy and counseling are very effective in processing the emotional responses of clients. Become skilled in the techniques and principles of or make referral to trained practitioners of the following methods: Gestalt, primal, bioenergetics, Reichian therapy, Radix work, or holotropic breathwork.

Previous mention has been made of the many psychologists and other mental healthcare professionals who recognize the connection between psychological states and physical states. When identifying and treating a neurosis, chemical addiction, or adjustment or relationship imbalances, they may recommend body therapies, such as deep tissue sculpting to increase awareness and reduce tension, as an adjunctive and concurrent therapy for their patients and clients.

Osteopathic Manipulative Treatment

Myofascial release and soft tissue manipulation are two of the treatment modalities employed by osteopathic physicians (DO) who manually treat their patients. While some osteopaths emphasize the importance of the soft tissue component in their treatment, for many this often is relegated to a few brief minutes of work preparatory to manipulation. Massage practitioners working with DOs are using deep tissue sculpting, especially in combination with deep cross-fiber friction, various neuromuscular techniques, and trigger point therapy. These integrated applications are performed prior to or concurrently with traditionally osteopathic treatments such as strain/counterstrain, muscle energy technique, and craniosacral therapy to provide maximum soft tissue release for the patient. The compatibility of sculpting and osteopathic manual treatment is high as there are many similarities and overlap between these soft tissue methodologies and deep tissue sculpting.

Chiropractic Healthcare

Deep tissue massage therapists working with chiropractors are powerful facilitators of chiropractic treatments. According to these therapists, sculpting reduces muscle spasm, fascial shortening, and generalized tension allowing for easier manipulations, more lasting adjustments, and decreased levels of tension for chiropractic patients. Many of these practitioners are integral members of chiropractors' staffs, treating their patients before and/or after adjustments; others work independently with clients who also enjoy these same benefits when receiving sculpting work concurrent with their chiropractic care.

Physicians and Other Healthcare Providers

Deep tissue sculpting is being used effectively by practitioners working with many physician specialists. This type of myofascial release facilitates recovery from reconstructive and other cosmetic surgeries. Orthopedic and sports medicine physicians often refer to or employ staff massage therapists to work with the myofascial components of various musculoskelal injuries and surgeries. Specific types of deep tissue sculpting relieve the prenatal and postpartum musculoskeletal discomforts obstetricians hear complaints of on a daily basis. Dentists treating temporomandibular joint dysfunctions (TMJ) also find sculpting work helpful in treating this often difficult-to-resolve condition.

Spas and Other Settings

Spas and resorts increasingly offer various massage and bodywork methodologies in addition to their "pampering" services of wraps, scrubs, and hydrotherapy. Deep tissue sculpting is an effective addition to the usual Swedish and relaxation massage techniques available in these facilities.

Sources Cited

[1] Fritz, Sandy. *Mosby's Fundamentals of Therapeutic Massage.* St. Louis, MO, Mosby Lifeline: 1995, pp. 80-81.

[2] For Trager bodywork, contact: Trager Institute, 21 Locust Avenue, Mill Valley, CA 94941. 415-388-2688. www.trager.com

[3] For passive joint movement and sensory repatterning bodywork, contact: James Stewart at International Professional School of Bodywork, 1366 Hornblend St., San Diego, CA 92128. 858-748-4142. www.IPSB.edu

[4] For movement coaching designed by Judith Aston, contact: Aston Training Center, P.O. Box 3568, Incline Village, NV 89450. 702-831-8228, www.aston-patterning.com Other movement systems such as Feldenkrais and Alexander also integrate well with sculpting.

[5] For rhythmic deep tissue (Blends) instruction, developed by Carole Osborne-Sheets, contact: Body Therapy Associates, 11650 Iberia Pl., #137, San Diego, CA 92128. 858-748-8827. www.bodytherapyassociates.com

[6] For stretching and ROM exercises to integrate with sculpting or to refer clients to trained practitioners, consult Bob Anderson, author of *Stretching*, Bolinas, CA, Shelter Publications, Inc.: 1980; Hanna Somatic Education, www.somaticsed.com; and Active Isolated Stretching, www.mattes.kudos.net

[7] For Rolf-based instruction and practitioners, contact: The Rolf Institute, www.rolf.org; Guild for Structural Integration, www.rolfguild.org; IPSB, www.IPSB.edu or www.anatomytrains.net

[8] Chaitow, DO, Leon. *Modern Neuromuscular Techniques.* Edinburgh, UK, Churchill Livingstone: 1996, p. 123.

[9] Maupin, Ph.D., Edward W. *The Genie in the Bottle: Psychology for Bodyworkers.* San Diego, CA: International Professional School of Bodywork, 1992, pp. 33-34.

[10] For integrative somatics specialization training, contact: IPSB at www.IPSB.edu

[11] For Rubenfeld Synergy trainings, contact: Rubenfeld Synergy Center at 212-315-3533.

[12] For Hakomi trainings, contact: Hakomi Institute at www.hakomiinstitute.com

[13] For trauma healing trainings, contact: Foundation for Human Enrichment at www.traumahealing.com

[14] For Upledger Institute courses, contact: The Uplegder Institute at www.upledger.com

[15] For John Barnes myofascial release seminars, contact: www.myofascialrelease.com

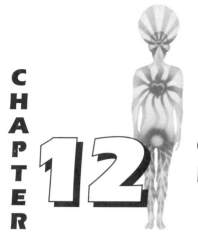

CHAPTER 12

Customizing Sculpting for Individual Clients

The three sessions of procedures detailed in Chapters Seven through Nine are designed to equip practitioners with techniques to address the most common complaints in general therapeutic massage and bodywork practices; however, unique individual clients have their own personal needs and concerns. This chapter offers guidance on how to respond in single sessions and session series to the particular needs of clients. Several focuses for organizing your work and example clients from actual practice will be discussed including:

- Complaint relief for soft tissue pain and tension
- Generalized chronic tension relief through balancing the three centers
- Structural balancing
- Retrieval and processing of emotions

Complaint Relief for Soft Tissue Pain and Tension

Most clients will detail one or several areas of pain, tension, or stiffness that has prompted them to seek the help of a bodywork practitioner. These complaints offer valuable clues for the design of appropriate therapy sessions. If the neck

hurts, sculpt there. A spasmed, painful anterior thigh needs stretching and sculpting of the quadriceps group. This approach attempts to relieve the presenting complaints, and does not primarily involve addressing underlying, contributing, or secondary imbalances. This primarily is the approach presented in the sessions detailed in this text. While this organizational method is the least inclusive, it is, in many cases, the quickest and easiest for you to implement. Rapid results can be achieved, though sometimes the relief is only temporary. For the most pervasive effects, be sure to consider all postural and movement clues, the client's overall balance, and the directly associated feelings.

Most simplistically, the client usually expects that the place that hurts will be touched. Some clients complain of impersonal doctors who never touched them for diagnosis or treatment. Others are frustrated by massage sessions for their sore arm or stiff neck when the practitioner, either by insight or misdirection, worked exclusively on some other area of the body, or did a general massage, allowing minimal time for the hurt area. The care of some of these practitioners may have been effective, while others will have completely missed the spot. In either case, most of their clients will feel that the innate human need and impulse to be touched where it hurts was not honored when the symptomatic part is not adequately and initially touched.

In addition to this psychological need, tactile input from the painful area can be invaluable to you in determining technique. Observe tissue texture and resistance, range and quality of motion, and localized and referred pain responses. Of course, the presenting area may not he the only site that requires sculpting and other therapeutic interventions.

An example client: "Alton"

Alton, a maintenance worker and carpenter for a major corporation, first came for relief from sharp pain in the left side of his neck. Extension of the cervical spine was particularly painful for him. He also reported pain in his left buttock and down into the back of his thigh, described by his chiropractor as sciatica. His first therapy session included work primarily from the neck and shoulder sculpting session and brief, rather superficial, sculpting of the gluteus medius and hamstring group. The image of lengthening the neck through a skyhook was explained, experienced, and suggested as a feeling to recreate frequently in his daily activities.

He reported feeling very stiff and sore for the first day following this session, then had dramatic improvement in his neck. While he seldom remembered to connect with his skyhook, when he did he reported feeling his neck noticeably more relaxed. His next session, one week after the first, was a repeat of the first session with additional emphasis on lengthening of the posterior fascial lines and relaxation of the erector spinae, gluteals, and the deep lateral rotators of the thigh. Several resisted stretches for these muscles were suggested and practiced.

One week later when he returned, Alton was still experiencing some sciatic pain, though greatly reduced. His neck had felt fine since his second session. A third session was primarily based on the low-back session, with additional work on the deep rotators once again. Passive and resisted assisted stretching of the gluteals, deep lateral rotators, hamstring group, and the gastrocnemius and soleus complex also were effective in completely relieving the sciatic symptoms.

Alton has continued for one year without sciatic pain, and has had only a few additional sessions, primarily in conjunction with a subsequent injury to his shoulder and arm.

Generalized Chronic Tension Relief Through Balancing the Three Centers

Focusing on balance of the three body centers (physical, emotional, and intellectual) effectively increases overall balance and helps to relieve generalized chronic tension. In a single session, reduce imbalance in the three centers by sculpting in the area of the most tension, and then draw freed energy to the center needing the most invigorating. Typically, clients have overcharged the intellectual center with work-related concerns and intellectualizations of living. The result: tension headaches, tight necks and shoulders, and a feeling of not existing below the head. Sculpt the neck, head, and shoulders to release this chronic tension and congestion. Then, use long sculpting strokes on the erector spinae. Sculpt the legs to connect them with the torso and to direct freed energy to the body areas connected with the physical center.

A series of three sessions can focus in turn on each of the three centers in whatever order is most appropriate for the client. Since the physical center is located three finger-widths below the navel and directly in the center of the lower abdomen, open and balance it through sculpting of the feet, legs, buttocks, and abdomen, with brief work in the back and neck to bring into awareness a connection with the other two centers. (Primarily procedures 7-10 and 13-l6 in the full body session, Chapter Ten, p. 112.)

In the second session of this series, attend to the feelings and the sense of relationship regulated through the heart center at the center of the chest. **(Image 58)** Emphasize sculpting and other work in the abdomen, chest, arms, and upper back in this session. (Procedures 5-7, and 11 in the full body session, Chapter Ten, pp. 111-112, and procedures 7,8,9 from the neck and shoulder session, Chapter Nine, pp. 107-108.) Again, include brief neck and feet work to bring in the other two centers.

Clear and balance the intellectual center, located between the eyebrows,

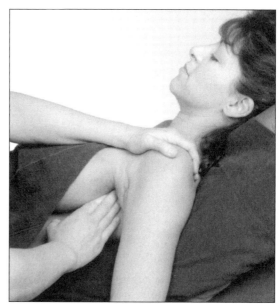

• **Image 58**: *Careful sculpting of the pectoralis minor helps to balance the pectoral girdle and normalize breath and feelings.*

with work that emphasizes release of the shoulders, neck, and head. (Procedure 4 in the full body session, Chapter Ten, p. 111, and most of the neck and shoulder session.) This final session, as in the two previously outlined, typically will include procedures that connect legs, arms, head, and torso, such as long effleurage strokes, hip and shoulder joint stretches, or rocking of the spine.

An example client: "Debbie"

While Debbie complained of neck and upper back stiffness, her primary interest was in achieving more clarity and balance in her life. A new, interracial romance was fulfilling, yet stressful for her. Her studies toward her doctorate were demanding. A three-centers approach felt more appropriate than dwelling on her neck and shoulder tension.

The first session primarily released her

chest, throat, and arms. As work in these areas proceeded, she cried as she remembered the anger and antagonism between her and her brother over their grandfather's affection. She tended to analyze the experience and block its intensity by intellectualizing. The session ended with discussion of the Jungian concepts of the internal male, the Animus, within each female.

Debbie's face, especially her jaws, and her neck were the focus of a second session. In contrast to the first, there was very little talking, and she cried briefly, yet profoundly.

Several weeks later, Debbie returned, reporting great improvement in her relationship, yet her finances were becoming shaky. This session then focused on her abdomen, legs, and the connection of her vitality to a solid base in the world. Exercises for generating and circulating energy were presented and practiced.

For several months, Debbie was seen monthly and continued exploring balance in her three centers, especially the emotional components of her tension. She felt that she was living in more harmony with all aspects of her Self. She had more energy and was less subject to extremely high or low moods. She also reported less neck and upper back stiffness.

Structural Balancing

For many clients, while discomfort may be felt, for example, in the low back, an underlying imbalance in the weight distribution in the feet or a change in the cervical spinal curvature is the key to long-term relief for the low back.

Ida Rolf's approach

In the mid-1960s, Ida Rolf, a biochemical engineer, began teaching a perspective and methodology for reorganizing the human structure, which she called Structural Integration, or Rolfing. Rolfing aims to configure the connective tissues into a more efficient, graceful, and energetic response to the primary force of gravity. Rolfers acknowledge alteration in fascial length and flexibility and its role of shaping the body's structure and determining the degree of functional structural balance. Put simply, in a series of 10 Rolfing sessions, the structure is adjusted to balance both vertical and horizontal polarities. Other geometric balances of the bisecting planes of the legs and arms, the side planes, and the transverse planes at the level of the shoulder, diaphragm, and pelvis are improved to produce more internal security and balance for the individual.[1] Rolfing is a comprehensive, effective system of deep tissue body therapy.[2]

Sculpting is quite similar to Rolfing and other forms of structural work (including Postural Integration, Hellerwork, and structural balancing) in the type of compressions, stroking, and holding of structures utilized. Sculpting, however, does not usually involve use of directed movement by the client to reorganize the fascia, a defining characteristic of Rolfing. (Ida Rolf's own summary of her approach was to "hold structures where they are supposed to be and induce movement."[3]) Additionally, in contrast to most of the aforementioned deep tissue methods, sculpting emphasizes the benefits of a very moderate pain and intensity level.

When seeking overall balance in the client's structural alignment, sculpt the entire body, facilitating release of the more extrinsic muscles of "doing," and then of the more intrinsic muscles of "being." (See p. 18 for a discussion of this distinction.) In general, work towards more balance between the body's "core" and its "sleeve."[4] Include some type of movement, as suggested in the previous chapter. (See pp. 118-120.)

Following the structural balancing guidelines first described by Ida Rolf[5] and further developed by Maupin[6], and others trained in this method, a minimum of 10 sculpting sessions is recommended for rebalancing structure. Design these sessions with focus on the following goals and areas to be addressed:

Session One

Goals To free the ribs and the pelvis from each other, to make breathing more effective, to make room in the torso for expansion of the organs, and to move the center of gravity to the physical center.

Areas to sculpt Chest, armpits, lateral torso and thigh, greater trocanter attachments, hamstring group, erector spinae, sternocleidomastoid (SCM), occipital ridge attachments.

Session Two

Goals To realign the ankle and knee more horizontally, to create a more solid connection with the ground through the legs, to lengthen the back.

Areas to sculpt Feet, anterior and lateral calves, erector spinae and associated fascial lines, SCM, occipital ridge attachments.

Session Three

Goals To lift the upper torso from the lumbar area, to free the twelfth rib, and create space for the quadratus lumborum.

Areas to sculpt Serratus anterior, latissimus dorsi, trapezius, rhomboids, erector spinae, teres major and minor, lumbodorsal fascia, quadratus lumborum, SCM, occipital ridge.

Session Four

Goals To release the pelvis, particularly the attachments at the ischium and pubis, to lengthen the adductors of the leg, to release the pelvic floor muscles, to continue horizontal balancing of the knee.

Areas to sculpt Medial sides of calves and thighs, ischial ramus, pubic bone, and coccyx attachments, erector spinae, SCM, occipital ridge attachments.

Session Five

Goals: To release the lumbar vertebrae, to release the iliopsoas, and to balance intrinsic and extrinsic (iliopsoas and abdominal) functions.

Areas to sculpt Abdominals, rib cage, diaphragm, iliopsoas, erector spinae, SCM, occipital ridge.

Session Six

Goals To release the rotators of the thigh, to organize the sacrum, and to release the posterior structures affecting pelvic alignment.

Areas to sculpt Posterior legs, ischial tuberosities, internal lateral rotators, sacrum and coccyx attachments, erector spinae, SCM, occipital ridge.

Session Seven

Goals To balance the head directly on the atlas vertebra, to release the cervical spine, to balance intrinsic and extrinsic muscle functions in the head and neck.

Areas to sculpt Attachments along the superior edge of the clavicle, facial muscles especially the masseter and temporalis, and fascial lines, temporomandibular joint, cervical facet joints, levator scapulae, supraspinatus, erector spinae, SCM, occipital ridge attachments.

Session Eight

Goals To create overall balance and energy flow in the pectoral girdle, and the arms.

Areas to sculpt Clavicle attachments (superior and inferior surfaces), pectoralis major and minor, rhomboids, anterior and posterior muscles of arms, hands, erector spinae, SMC, occipital ridge attachments.

Session Nine

Goals To create overall balance and energy flow through the pelvis, to balance movement in the hip joint, to establish the pelvis as a reliable and resilient structure for weight bearing, to relieve the upper torso, neck, and head for upward extension.

Areas to sculpt All attachments on the pelvis, especially the intrinsic muscles (quadratus lumborum, lateral rotators, iliopsoas, pelvic floor), erector spinae, SMC, occipital ridge attachments.

Session Ten and Beyond

Goals To integrate the structure toward vertical alignment; horizontal alignment of ankle, knees, anterior superior iliac spines, clavicles and eyes; frontal plane alignment of the pelvis and shoulders; to facilitate a sense of a balanced polarity of energy movement upward and downward; to elongate and decompress all myofascia and joints.

Areas to sculpt Whatever still needs release.

Myers' myofascial meridians

Although he has practiced and taught Rolf's method of Structural Integration for over 25 years, only recently has Tom Myers elegantly articulated his unique and engaging view of structural integration and balance. Using the metaphor of railway or train lines, he illustrates and describes holistic interconnected paths among the muscles, bones, and their myofascial network. He has identified these anatomy trains, or myofascial meridians, winding throughout the body and creating a scaffold of tensional bands and bony spacers that make up the unique skeletal sculpture of individuals. Some examples of these meridians are the superficial back and front lines and the spiral line.[7] Although elaboration of his principles for treatment following these lines is beyond the scope of this manual, this gifted, inspiring teacher's writings and instructional programs are highly recommended.[8]

An example client: "Casey"

The first four sessions on Casey, a retired naval officer working on a doctorate in computer education, were directed toward relief of the chronic tension she experienced in her neck and shoulders. She also was experiencing sciatic pain, which periodically flared up to make her quite uncomfortable. In the two months during which these sessions were scheduled, she also began counseling with a therapist as a continuation of her recovery from alcoholism.

While the initial work relieved the sciatic pain, Casey expressed concern that she did not want to be plagued with recurring bouts of sciatica, and the relief from her neck and shoulder tension was not long-lasting enough. An overall

structural approach to her body seemed appropriate to facilitate more lasting relief.

Over the next six months, bimonthly work proceeded through the session series outlined above. Interspersed with these structurally oriented sessions were other symptomatic work when appropriate: a soothing, relaxing massage after a tax audit; inner thigh and consensual pelvic floor attachment work (externally applied) coinciding with processing of sexual issues in her therapy sessions. Free of sciatic pain and most chronic neck and shoulder tension, Casey continues to receive sculpting and other integrative bodywork monthly for health maintenance.

Retrieval and Processing of Emotions

Mom's arms embrace baby welcoming him to the family. She and father gently count all the toes: "This little piggy went to market...." Soon a toddler, his bedtime usually means back rubs, and when his brow is fevered, he is soothed with soft strokes. Later, understanding hugs acknowledge his teenage successes or failures, and he and his family treat his rapidly maturing body with respect and love.

Nourishing families supply their members with touch that conveys assurance, pleasure, warmth, vitality and self-esteem. Nurturing touch is a natural part of a healthy, functioning family unit. The children of alcoholic and other dysfunctional families, however, often grow up experiencing primarily abusive touch such as violent beatings, sexual abuse, or physical or emotional neglect.

Children of alcoholics, other substance abusers, and dysfunctional families often experience a childhood environment of uncertainty, chaos, and pain. Emotional, and sometimes physical, abandonment, hurt, and shame characterize their family life. Many experience one or a series of catastrophic events that are not resolved either physically or psychologically, leaving them in a state of chronic shock.[9]

While there probably are some good times, basically these children survive by their own internal protection system. The child of a dysfunctional family must construct a physical, emotional, intellectual, and spiritual fortress as the only stronghold in the chaotic landscape of his life. Within, the wounded child hides, usually continuing into adult life feeling increasingly alone, hollow, and aching, and only able to temporarily numb himself with activities or substances. Some psychologists refer to these individuals as Adult Children of Alcoholics (ACAs).[10]

Their fortress typically is physically constructed of tight muscles, particularly in the neck, shoulders and lower back, sexual and gastrointestinal dysfunction, and allergies. Its walls often are emotionally reinforced by distrust, fear, anger, sadness, numbness, or overly aggressive or overly passive behavior. Many are unable to distinguish loving healthy touch from aggression and abuse. Within these protective walls, the individual is not only isolated from his dysfunctional family, but also becomes divorced from his own sense of Self. Connection with his own body and feelings is broken. Boundaries and limits within relationships are often ill-defined as well.

Sculpting and emotional processing

When a client feels ready to break down the walls of his old defenses, therapeutic massage, particularly deep tissue sculpting, can provide a safe context for change. Appropriate hands-on therapy can decrease muscle tension and increase body awareness. In a professional setting of touch and sensory input, issues of touch, trust, intimacy, and communication arise. Opportunities to explore healthy personal boundaries are inherent in the relationship. Knowing, loving, nonintrusive touch can facilitate the recovery and release of traumatic memories buried in the body's defenses. Clients can investigate more nurturing ways of touching and being touched and learn to incorporate these skills into a new, more mature sense of Self. Of course, many clients also need the care of a psychologist or counselor.

Many clients from dysfunctional families come to process, recover, and rest on body therapy tables. Some initially seek relief from injury, chronic tension, or pain. Some just want to relax and escape the stress of their lives. Increasing numbers of psychologists and other mental healthcare providers recognize massage therapy and other somatic therapies as very direct approaches to the locked body and feelings of some of their patients. Much inspiring personal growth and healing occurs in therapeutic bodywork practices, while the unresolved struggle of other clients is sometimes the undesired, but unavoidable reality.

Many individuals come from inflexible

families that were unable to adapt to change easily or willingly. To create and maintain this rigidity, their bodies themselves become inflexible. Tense neck, shoulder, and back muscles are common. Tension in these areas is necessary in a subconscious attempt to control the chaos of the dysfunctional family system. These clients' spinal and pelvic joints are especially limited and rigid in quantity and quality of movement. Their gait is often disjointed, arrhythmic, or lacking in grace and fluidity.

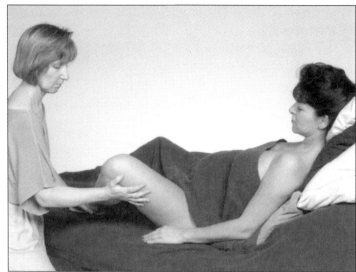

• **Image 59**: *Low amplitude, slow rhythmic movements combine well with sculpting to restore physical and emotional flexibility.*

Use fluid, rhythmical, passive rocking and shaking movements to help soften this controlling rigidity. **(Image 59)** To bring more flexibility to the body, assist in stretching tight muscles. Sculpt on knotted, hard muscle and fascia to soften the physical rigidity. On an emotional level, sculpting will encourage the need to control to give way to more spontaneity in expression. Playfulness and real happiness then becomes more possible.

The dysfunctional family does not freely talk about what is happening in the family either with its members or others. In fact, talking about any feelings is usually avoided. Thus the fear, anger, and hurt with which the individual has grown up, are usually very difficult to cope with and are repressed.

As the soft tissue of the body undergoing sculpting begins to yield some of its rigidity, encourage a corresponding change on the emotional level. Be open to long-suppressed feeling exploding in angry tirades, slipping to the surface in sighs and groans, or flooding tears. In the trusting intimacy of a bodywork session, feelings and traumatic incidents can be explored, expressed, and resolved. Facilitate closure and resolution when these types of memories surface by using interior dialogue techniques and creative visualizations. Be prepared to refer those who need psychological services to counselors and therapists.

Many individuals live for years with denial that there was an alcohol problem or other problems in their family. As children, they were taught to deny what their eyes showed them, their ears told them, and their hearts felt. Thus, a tremendous conflict can develop between what the child saw and felt and what he was told was occurring. Denial of his own feelings and lack of trust in his body awareness are the usual outcomes of this familial conflict.

The immediacy, intimacy, and sensory reality of body therapy can directly challenge many clients to feel, and feel intensely. The immense tactile input of the stroking, kneading, and percussion movements of Swedish massage is often effective in overwhelming these denial mechanisms. As his skin and muscles are rhythmically rubbed and milked, not only are blood and lymph circulated, but the client also begins to take notice of his body's messages. To move deeply into expressing emotion, sculpting in conjunction with interior dialogue techniques, bioenergetics, guided fantasy and breathing, and movement and sensory awareness exercises are effective. (See Chapter Four, pp. 47-56.)

An example client: "Sarah"

Sarah had been in counseling for several months when she first sought massage therapy for tension in her neck and back. She said that she felt generally numb. She and her counselor hoped that she could release the physical and emotional tension that she retained. She also wanted to learn from the inside when touch and intimacy are safe. She told, in a rather detached manner, several childhood stories of sexual and emotional abuse in her alcoholic, dysfunctional family.

On the table, Sarah vigilantly kept her eyes open and alert to every move. When tight areas of her back and neck were kneaded and stroked, she began to experience herself as a little girl alone and sad. When deeper compressions uncovered painful spots, she

acknowledged that she could numb herself to any pain she felt. Then she discovered that if she relaxed and observed, the muscle began to soften, and pain transformed into awareness. What an empowering, undeniably real lesson!

Touch can bring to consciousness what can be hidden in thoughts and words. Over the weeks of her body therapy, she sometimes graphically recalled abusive, traumatic incidents in her early life. Initially, the memories would intensify the rigidity in Sarah's back and neck, as well as the generalized lack of awareness in her body, especially in her legs. With encouragement and direction, she was able to express the associated unresolved feelings and actions of those events. Though she had talked about all of this before, now she sometimes cried, fought, and yelled. She knew in a more tangible way not only the trauma, but also the necessary defenses her body and heart put up. Her body awareness and her sensitivity to her feelings began to increase dramatically.

Soon, the subtle rocking and shaking movements of her legs, which were blended with the sculpting, were more than a challenge to her protective fortress. Sometimes she could feel the pleasure of kinesthetic awareness in allowing her hip and leg to be passively floated through their range of motion. The tightness in her shoulders was softening, and, as the muscles melted from their chronic tension, she felt delicious relief.

Sometimes Sarah requested relaxing circulatory massage for an enjoyable, nurturing reward for her progress. Her sense of her Self, physically and emotionally, was strengthening. She came to know and trust that touch can be respectful, knowledgeable, and loving. That positive experience then helped to generate more trusting, expansive movement in her life.

Outside of therapy sessions and off the massage table, she started to live in a more adult, internally successful way. She had always been "functional;" she was an effective labor and delivery nurse, but now she enrolled in classes for the counseling career she wanted to pursue. A series of incompatible roommates was broken by a woman who became her friend. Eventually, she entered into a healthy relationship with a man, a need that had both enticed and totally terrified her previously. As she completed a year and a half of bimonthly work, she learned to erect a fortress in her body and emotions when she needed protection, and dissolve it when not.

Another example client: "Lori"

Lori, a 29-year-old woman, originally came seeking relief from chronic neck and shoulder pain, which recently had increased to acute severity while doing bench presses. She had been in two auto accidents two years prior, and in the last one she had overturned her car and hit her head on the car ceiling. She suffered bilateral pain, tightness, and limited range of motion in her neck, but more severely on the left side. She had received chiropractic treatment from which she had initially had some positive effect. She reported no other major injuries or illnesses, present or past. Labeling herself

as an introvert, she explained that her work as a financial advisor involved significant interaction with clientele, and she no longer found much satisfaction in her work.

An osteopathic physician's evaluation revealed considerable myofascial restriction in the cervical and thoracic areas, as well as restriction in their movement. The diagnosis was cervical and upper back sprain and somatic dysfunction of the cervical and thoracic regions. Structural observations prior to beginning body therapy revealed some increased lumbar curvature, elevation of the shoulders with the left shoulder higher and anteriorly rotated, a tilt of the head toward the left and down, compression in the cervical vertebrae, and a winging out of both scapulae. Range of movement of her neck decreased markedly in rotation, particularly to the left, in lateral flexion to the left, and in extension.

Weekly sessions with Lori involved extensive deep tissue sculpting, blended with passive joint movements, as well as cross-fiber friction, strain/counterstrain, and structural balancing. Immediate relief of most pain lasted for several consecutive days between sessions, then tightness would set in again and the pain would return, though never with its initial severity.

Six months into her therapy, Lori shared that she had a novel inside her that she longed to write. She felt trapped in her job, however, with little time or energy left with which to write. She also had been doing some reading in body/mind literature, and wondered if perhaps there were some unresolved emotions hindering a more complete recovery from her injuries. As her neck was sculpted during the next session, she began remembering the auto accident and the sensation of being out of control: in the careening car, in excesses in her personal life, in overworking but being dissatisfied. Her recall of the events and feelings of the accident guided her into the rage she felt at her job and at the car that got her around in her job, and the deep wish that they both be smashed into a million pieces. As she concluded her memory, she uncovered her guilt that although she had been "living so badly," strangers at a nearby house were very kind to her immediately after the accident.

Two weeks later, Lori reported that her neck was greatly improved and had remained mostly pain-free. She also had started writing her novel, and had figured out how to responsibly quit her job so that she could continue writing and support herself. She was feeling free and alive. Subsequent, less frequent sessions of deep tissue sculpting and other therapeutic bodywork have helped her to maintain continued improvement in her neck, though she has had a few minor regressions to increased pain.

Sources Cited

[1] Maupin, Ph.D., Edward W. *The Structural Metaphor: An Introduction to the Rolf Method of Structural Integration*, Part I, 2001, pp.8-15.

[2] Cottingham, John T. *Healing through Touch: A History and a Review of the Physiological Evidence*. Boulder, CO: Rolf Institute, 1985.

[3] Maupin, Op. Cit., p.9.

[4] Maupin, Op. Cit., p.11.

[5] Rolf, Ida P. *Rolfing: The Integration of Human Structures*. New York, NY: Harper and Row, 1977.

[6] Maupin, Op. Cit. and Part II of same publication.

[7] Myers, Thomas W. *The Anatomy Trains; Myofascial Meridians for Manual and Movement Therapists*. Edinburgh, UK: Churchill Livingstone, 2001.

[8] For Kinesis Myofascial Integration school information, contact: Kinesis Seminars, Inc. at www.anatomytrains.net

[9] Kritsberg, Wayne. *The Adult Children of Alcoholics Syndrome, From Discovery to Recovery*. New York, NY: Bantam Books, 1988, pp. 15-31.

[10] Bradshaw, John. Bradshaw on: *The Family. A Revolutionary Way of Self-Discovery*. Deerfield Beach, FL: Health Communications, Inc.,

In Conclusion:
Coming Full Circle

While the written word, illustrations, and photographs are relevant means of teaching, their limitations are obvious in communicating the feel of sculpting. Coursework and individualized instruction provide the essential hands-on, personal experience of the work.

Studying this manual launches you into the process of acquiring experience in the use of deep tissue sculpting. Extend your study and experience by integrating and improvising on the many applications to which sculpting lends itself. It is this sort of utilization and personalizing of technique that will make deep tissue sculpting not only a powerful therapeutic modality but also your own artistic expression.

It has been the intention of this manual to provide students and practitioners with thorough instruction in both the technical, factual aspects and the affective and artistic qualities of deep tissue sculpting. Throughout, emphasis has been on balance: balance of structure, of yin/yang energies, and of physical and somato-emotional applications of the work.

May each practitioner seriously study all that has been offered: the technique, the anatomy, the indications and contraindications, the psychological associations, and the guidance in body mechanics. Then, with equal dedication and fervor, may you allow pure love, intuition, artistic style, and clarity of spirit to guide and to inspire your work, for the benefit of all Humanity and the realization of Humanity One.

SUPPLEMENTING

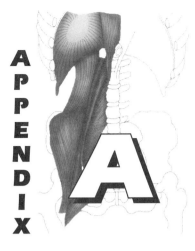

APPENDIX A

Muscular Anatomy Relevant to Sculpting Sessions

BICEPS BRACHII

Origin   Short head: coracoid process of scapula

Long head: supraglenoid tubercle of scapula

Insertion   Tuberosity of radius and aponeurosis of the biceps brachii

Function   Flexion of elbow

Supination of forearm

Short head: flexion of humerus

BICEPS FEMORIS

Origin   Long head: ischial tuberosity

Short head: Lateral lip of linea aspera

Insertion   Head of fibula

Function   Long head: extension of hip

Both heads: flexion of knee, lateral rotation of hip and flexed knee

Tilt pelvis posteriorly

DELTOIDS

Origin   Anterior: lateral third of clavicle

Middle: lateral acromion

Posterior: spine of scapula

Insertion   Deltoid tuberosity of humerus

Function   Anterior: flexion, horizontal adduction, medial rotation of humerus

Middle: abduction of humerus to 90^0

Posterior: extension, horizontal abduction, lateral rotation of humerus

ERECTOR SPINAE GROUP
Origin   Common tendon (thorocolumbar aponeurosis) that attaches to posterior surface of sacrum, iliac crest, spinous processes of the lumbar and last two thoracic vertebrae

Insertion   Various attachments at posterior ribs, spinous and transverse processes of thoracic and cervical vertebrae, mastoid process of temporal bone

Function   Action bilaterally: extend vertebral column unilaterally
Laterally: flex vertebral column to same side

EXTERNAL OBLIQUE ABDOMINAL
Origin   Lower eight ribs

Insertion   Abdominal aponeurosis and anterior iliac crest

Function   Bilaterally: flexion of trunk, compression of abdominal contents
Unilaterally: lateral flexion, rotation of trunk to opposite side

GLUTEUS MAXIMUS
Origin   Posterior sacrum, posterior iliac crest, sacrotuberous and sacroiliac ligaments

Insertion   Gluteal tuberosity of femur and iliotibial tract (which continues to attach to lateral condyle of tibia)

Function   Forceful extension of hip, lateral rotation of extended hip, lower fibers adduct hip

GLUTEUS MEDIUS
Origin   External surface of the ilium between iliac crest and posterior and anterior gluteal line

Insertion   Greater trochanter of femur

Function   Abduction, medial and lateral rotation of hip, flexion and extension of hip

GLUTEUS MINIMUS
Origin   Exterior ilium between anterior and inferior gluteal lines

Insertion   Anterior surface of greater trochanter of femur

Function   Abduction, medial rotation of hip

HAND AND FINGER EXTENSORS
Origin   Mostly lateral epicondyle

Insertion   Mostly the metacarpals

Function   Extension of the wrist and fingers

HAND AND FINGER FLEXORS

Origins Primarily on the medial epicondyle of the humerus and on the radius, ulna and interosseous membranes between these bones
Insertions Primarily on the posterior surface of the carpals, metacarpals, and phalanges
Functions Flexion of the wrist and fingers

INTERNAL OBLIQUE ABDOMINAL

Origin Inguinal ligament and anterior iliac crest, thoracolumbar fascia
Insertion Costal cartilages of last three ribs
Abdominal aponeurosis
Function Bilaterally: flexion of thorax, compression of abdominal contents
Unilaterally: lateral flexion, rotation of trunk to same side

LATISSIMUS DORSI

Origin Thoracolumbar aponeurosis and posterior iliac crest, lower three or four ribs, spinous processes of last six thoracic vertebrae
Insertion Crest of the lesser tubercle of humerus
Function Extension, medial rotation and adduction of humerus

LEVATOR SCAPULA

Origin C-1 to C-4 (transverse processes)
Insertion Vertebral border of scapula from superior angle to root of spine of scapula
Function Elevation of scapula, downward rotation of scapula, lateral flexion of neck and head

PECTORALIS MAJOR

Origin Clavicular head: medial half of clavicle
Sternal head: sternum, cartilages of upper six ribs
Insertion Lateral lip bicipital groove of humerus
Function Generally adduction, horizontal adduction and medial rotation of humerus
Clavicular head: flexion of humerus
Sternal head: extension of humerus from a flexed position

PSOAS MAJOR AND ILIACUS

Origin Psoas major: lumbar vertebrae
Iliacus: inner surface of ilium
Insertion Lesser trochanter of femur
Function Flexion, adduction, and lateral rotation of hip

QUADRATUS LUMBORUM
Origin   Posterior iliac crest
Insertion   12th rib, transverse processes of lumbar vertebrae
Function   Lateral flexion of trunk or raises hip

RECTUS ABDOMINUS
Origin   Pubis symphasis
Insertion   Costal cartilages 5, 6, 7
Function   Flexion of trunk, compression of abdominal contents

RECTUS FEMORIS
Origin   Anterior inferior iliac spine, upper margin of acetabulum
Insertion   Patella and via patellar ligament to tibial tuberosity
Function   Extension of knee, assists flexion of hip

RHOMBOIDS: MAJOR AND MINOR
Origin   Minor: C-7 and T-1 (spinous processes)
                   Major: T-2 to T-5 (spinous processes)
Insertion   Minor: root of spine of scapula
                   Major: vertebral border of scapula from root of spine to inferior angle
Function   Retract, elevate, downward rotate scapula

SCALENES: ANTERIOR, MEDIUS, AND POSTERIOR
Origin   Transverse processes of cervical vertebrae
Insertion   First two ribs (anterior and medius to first rib; posterior to second rib)
Function   Bilaterally: raise first two ribs during forced inspiration or assist neck flexion
                   Unilaterally: assist in lateral flexion to same side, rotate neck to opposite side

SEMIMEMBRANOSUS AND SEMITENDINOSUS
Origin   Ischial tuberosity
Insertion   Semimembranosus: Posterior medial tibial condyle
                   Semitendinosus: Anterior proximal tibial shaft
Function   Extension of hip, flexion of knee, medial rotation of flexed knee

SPLENIUS CAPITIS AND CERVICIS
Origin   Splenius capitis: Ligamentum nuchae, spinous processes lower cervical
                   vertebra (C-7), spinous processes upper thoracic vertebrae (T-1 to T-3)
                   Splenius cervicis: Spinous processes upper thoracic vertebrae (T-3 to T-6)
Insertion   Splenius capitis: Mastoid process and occipital bone
                   Splenius cervicis: Upper cervical vertebrae (transverse processes C-1 to C-3)

Function   Bilaterally: extension of head

                 Unilaterally: rotation of head to same side, laterally flex head and neck

STERNOCLEIDOMASTOID (SCM)
Origin   Manubrium of sternum, medial clavicle
Insertion   Mastoid process
Function   Bilaterally: flexion of neck

                 Unilaterally: lateral flexion, rotation of head to opposite side

SUBOCCIPITALS
Origin   Atlas and axis vertebrae
Insertion   Nuchal line of occiput, between nuchal lines and transverse process of atlas
Function   Rock and tilt head back into extension; rotate head to same side

SUPRASPINATUS
Origin   Supraspinous fosoa of scapula
Insertion   Greater tubercle of humerus
Function   Abducts humerus

                 Stabilizes head of humerus in glenoid cavity

TERES MAJOR
Origin   Inferior angle of scapula
Insertion   Medial lip of bicipital groove of humerus
Function   Extension, medial rotation and adduction of humerus

TERES MINOR
Origin   Upper axillary border of scapula
Insertion   Greater tubercle of humerus
Function   Lateral rotation, extension of humerus

TRANSVERSE ABDOMINUS
Origin   Inguinal ligament, iliac crest, thoracolumbar aponeurosis, lower margin

                 of rib cage
Insertion   Abdominal aponeurosis and linea alba, pubis
Function   Compression of abdominal contents

TRAPEZIUS
Origin   Occiput, ligamentum nuchae C-7 to T-12 (spinous processes)
Insertion   Upper: lateral clavicle, acromion

                 Middle: spine of scapula

Function   Lower: root of spine of scapula
Upper: elevation, forward rotation of scapula
Middle: adduction and stabilization of scapula
Lower: depression, upward rotation of scapula

TRICEPS BRACHII AND ANCONEUS

Origin   Long head: infraglenoid tubercle of scapula
Lateral head: posterior humerus above spiral groove
Medial head: posterior humerus below spiral groove
Insertion   Olecranon process of ulna
Function   Extension of elbow
Long head: extension, adduction of humerus

VASTUS MEDIALIS, LATERALIS, AND INTERMEDIUS

Origin   Vastus medialis: medial lip of linea aspera on posterior femur
Vastus lateralis: lateral lip of linea aspera on posterior femur
Vastus intermedius: anterior and lateral femoral shaft
Insertion   Patella and via patellar ligament to tibial tuberosity
Function   Extension of knee

Source for this Outline:
Biel, Andrew. *Trail Guide to the Body: How to locate muscles, bones and more.* Boulder, CO: Andrew Biel, 1997

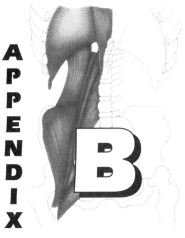

B Skeletal Anatomy Relevant to Sculpting Sessions

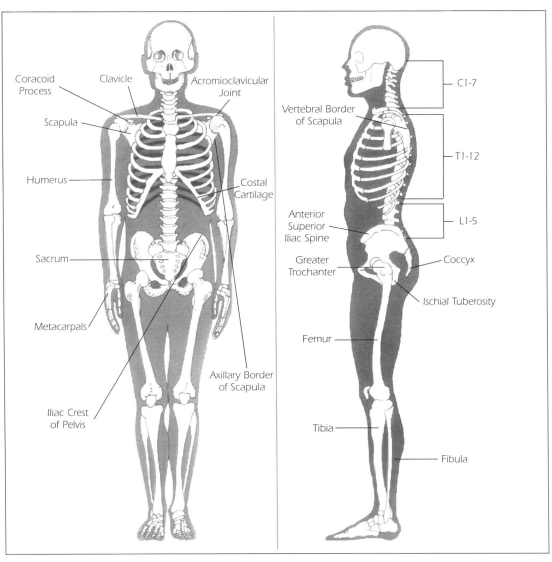

Coracoid Process
Clavicle
Acromioclavicular Joint
Scapula
Humerus
Costal Cartilage
Sacrum
Metacarpals
Iliac Crest of Pelvis
Axillary Border of Scapula

C1-7
Vertebral Border of Scapula
T1-12
Anterior Superior Iliac Spine
L1-5
Greater Trochanter
Coccyx
Ischial Tuberosity
Femur
Tibia
Fibula

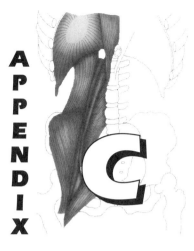

Bibliography

Anderson, Bob. *Stretching.* Bolinas, CA: Shelter Publications Inc. 1980.

Barnes, John F. *Healing Ancient Wounds: The Renegade's Wisdom.* Paoli, PA: Rehabilitation Services, Inc. 2000.

_____ "The Myofascial Release: Mind/Body Healing Approach," *Massage Magazine* (January/February, 1998): 91-94.

Barnes, Mark F. "The Basic Science of Myofascial Release: Morphologic change in connective tissue." *Journal of Bodywork and Movement Therapies* (July 1997): 231-238.

Basmajian, John V., M.D. *Muscles Alive.* Baltimore, MD: The Williams and Wilkins Co. 1967.

_____. *Primary Anatomy.* Baltimore, MD: The Williams and Wilkins Co. 1970.

Beck, Mark. *The Theory and Practice of Therapeutic Massage.* Bronx, NY: Milady Publishing Inc. 1988.

Benjamin, Ben. *Are You Tense?* New York, NY: Pantheon Books. 1978.

Benjamin, Ben with Gale Borden, M.D. *Listen to Your Pain.* New York, NY: Penguin Books. 1984.

Biel, Andrew. *Trail Guide to the Body.* Boulder, CO: Andrew Biel. 1997.

"Body and Soul". *Newsweek* (November 7, 1988): 88-90.

Bradshaw, John. *Bradshaw on: The Family. A Revolutionary Way of Self-Discovery.* Deerfield Beach, FL: Health Communications, Inc. 1988.

Cailliet, Rene, M.D. *Soft Tissue Pain and Disability.* Philadelphia, PA: F.A. Davis Co. 1977.

Calais-Germain, Blandine. *Anatomy of Movement.* Seattle, WA: Eastland Press. 1993.

Calvert, Robert. "Exclusive Interview with Dr. Milton Trager." *Massage Magazine 15* (August/September 1988): 12-32.

Carver, Claudia. "Sensitive Treatment for Survivors of Childhood Sexual Abuse." *Massage Magazine* (Jan/Feb 2001): 171-178.

SUPPLEMENTING...

Chaitow, Leon, N.D., D.O. *Modern Neuromuscular Techniques.* Edinburgh, Scotland: Churchill Livingstone. 1996.

Cottingham, John T. *Healing through Touch: A History and a Review of the Physiological Evidence.* Boulder, CO: Rolf Institute. 1985.

Coulter, Harris L. *Divided Legacy: The Conflict Between Homeopathy and the American Medical Association. Science and Ethics in American Medicine*, 1800-1914, Volume III. Richmond, CA: North Atlantic Books. 1982.

Curties, Debra. *Massage Therapy and Cancer.* New Brunswick, Canada: Curties-Overzet Publications, Inc. 1999.

Dicke, E., H. Schliack, A. Wolff. *A Manual of Reflexive Therapy of the Connective Tissue (Connective Tissue Massage)* "Bindegewebsmassage." Scarsdale, NY: Sidney S. Simon. 1978.

Drury, Nevill. *The Bodywork Book.* Dorset, England: Prism Alpha. 1984.

Dychtwald, Ken. *Bodymind.* Los Angeles, CA: Tarcher. 1986.

Eisenberg, et. al. "Trends in Alternative Medicine Use in the United States, 1990-1997." *Journal of the American Medical Association*, 280(18): November 11, 1998: 1569-1575.

Feitis, Rosemary, Editor. *Ida Rolf Talks About Rolfing and Physical Reality.* New York, NY: Harper and Row. 1978.

Field, T., M. Hernandez-Rief, S. Hart, et al. "Pregnant women benefit from massage therapy." *Journal of Psychosomatic Obstetrics and Gynecology.* (March, 1999) 20(1): 31-38.

Ford, Clyde. *Compassionate Touch.* Park Ridge, IL: Parkside Publishing. 1993.

Fritz, Sandy. *Mosby's Fundamentals of Therapeutic Massage.* St. Louis, MO: Mosby-Year Book, Inc. 1995.

Galante, Laurence. *Tai Chi the Supreme Ultimate.* York Beach, ME: Samuel Weiser, Inc. 1981.

Guinness, Alma E., editor. *Family Guide to Natural Medicine.* Pleasantwille, NY: Reader's Digest Association, Inc. 1993.

Hanna, Thomas. *Somatics.* Reading, MA: Addison-Wesley Publishing Co. Inc. 1988.

Hoppenfield, Stanley, M.D. *Physical Examination of the Spine and Extremities.* New York, NY: Appleton-Century Crofts. 1976.

Ichazo, Oscar. *Psychocalisthenics.* New York, NY: Simon and Schuster. 1976.

Jacobs, Miriam. "Massage for the relief of pain: anatomical and physiological considerations." *Physical Therapy Review* (June, 1959): 93-98.

Juhan, Deane. *Job's Body: A Handbook for Bodywork, Expanded Edition.* New York, NY: Station Hill Press. 1998.

Keen, Sam. "We have no desire to strengthen the ego or make it happy," an interview with Oscar Ichazo. *Psychology Today* (July, 1973):

Keleman, Stanley. *Emotional Anatomy.* Berkeley, CA: Center Press. 1985.

Koch, Liz. *The Psoas Book* (second edition). Felton, CA: Guinea Pig Publications. 1997.

Kritsberg, Wayne. *The Adult Children of Alcoholics Syndrome, From Discovery to Recovery.* New York, NY: Bantam Books. 1988.

Kurtz, Ron. *Body-Centered Psychotherapy: The Hakomi Method.* Mendocino, CA: LifeRhythm. 1990.

Kurtz, Ron, and Hector Prestera. *The Body Reveals.* New York, NY: Harper and Row. 1976.

Levine, Peter with Ann Frederick. *Waking the Tiger: Healing Trauma.* Berkeley, CA: North Atlantic Books. 1997.

MacDonald, Gayle. *Medicine Hands: Massage Therapy for People with Cancer.* Forres, Scotland: Findhorn Press. 1999.

Maupin, Edward W. *The Genie in the Bottle: Psychology for Bodyworkers.* San Diego, CA: International Professional School of Bodywork. 1992.

——————————. *The Structural Metaphor.* San Diego, CA: International Professional School of Bodywork. 2001.

McNeely, Deldon Anne. *Touching: Body Therapy and Depth Psychology.* Toronto, Canada: Inner City Books. 1987.

Mower, Melissa B. "The Team Approach to a Body/Mind Session." *Massage Magazine 71* (Jan-Feb., 1998): 32-39.

Myers, Thomas W. *Anatomy Trains: Myofascial Meridians for Manual and Movement Therapists.* London, UK : Churchill Livingstone. 2001.

——————————. "Body Cubed" (article series). *Massage Magazine* Issues (September/October, 1997-January/February. 2000).

——————————. "The Anatomy Trains." *Journal of Bodywork and Movement Therapies*: 1(2), January, 1997: 94.

Osborne-Sheets, Carole. *Pre- and Perinatal Massage Therapy.* San Diego, CA: Body Therapy Associates. 1998.

Oschman, Jim. "What is Healing Energy? Part 5: Gravity, Structure, and Emotions." *Journal of Bodywork and Movement Therapies* (October, 1997).

Ostgaard, H.C., Andersson, G.B.S., et al. "Prevalence of back pain in pregnancy." *Spine* January 1992, 17(1): 53-55.

Pert, Candace B. *Molecules of Emotion.* New York, NY: Scribner. 1997.

Premkumar, Kalyani. *Pathology A to Z: a Handbook for Massage Therapists.* Calgary, AB, Canada: VanPub Books. 1996.

Reich, Wilhelm. *The Function of the Orgasm.* New York, NY: World Publishing. 1942.

Rolf, Ida. *Rolfing: The Integration of Human Structures.* New York, NY: Harper and Row. 1977.

Rose, Colin and Malcolm J. Nicholl. *Accelerated Learning for the 21st Century.* New York, NY: Delacorte Press. 1997.

Rosse, Cornelius, M.D., and D. Kay Clawson, M.D. *The Musculoskeletal System in Health and Disease.* New York, NY: Harper and Row. 1980.

SUPPLEMENTING...

Smolen, Rick, Phillip Moffitt, and Matthew Naythons, M.D. *The Power to Heal: Ancient Arts and Modern Medicine.* New York, NY: Prentice Hall Press. 1990.

Snyder, George E. "Fasciae-Applied Anatomy and Physiology." *Journal of the American Osteopathic Association,* March, 1969, 68.

Southmayd, William, M.D., and Marshall Hoffman. *Sportshealth. The Complete Book of Athletic Injuries.* New York, NY: Quick Fox. 1981.

Stanford University School of Medicine. "Complementary and Alternative Medicine: Scientific Evidence and Steps Towards Integration." Conference held September, 1999.

Starlanyl, Devin, M.D. and Mary Ellen Copeland. *Fibromyalgia and Chronic Myofascial Pain Syndrome.* Oakland, CA: New Harbinger Publications, Inc. 1996.

"Tai Chi for Health" (video). Venice, CA: Healing Arts Publishing Inc. 800-2-LIVING

Tappan, Frances M. *Healing Massage Techniques: Holistic, Classic, and Emerging Methods.* USA: Appleton and Lange. 1988.

Timms, Robert and Patrick Connors. *Embodying Healing: Integrating Bodywork and Psychotherapy in Recovery from Childhood Sexual Abuse.* Orwell, VT: Safer Society Press. 1992.

Travell, Janet G., M.D. and David G. Simons, M.D. *Myofascial Pain and Dysfunction, Volumes One and Two.* Baltimore, MD: Williams and Wilkins. 1992.

Twomley L., J. Taylor. "Flexion, Creep, Dysfunction and Hysteresis in the Lumbar Vertebral Column," *Spine 7,2* (1982): 116-122.

Upledger, John E., D.O., and Jon D. Vredevoogd. *Craniosacral Therapy.* Seattle, WA: Eastland Press. 1983.

van der Giessen, Matthew J. "Psyche and Soma," *Massage Therapy Journal.* (Summer, 1990): 67-72.

Vickers, Andrew. *Massage and Aromatherapy: A Guide for Health Professionals.* London, UK: Chapman and Hall. 1996.

Walton, Tracy. "Clinical Thinking and Cancer." *Massage Therapy Journal.* (Fall, 2000): 66-80.

Weil, Andrew, M.D. *Spontaneous Healing.* New York, NY: Ballantine Books. 1995.

Yates, John. *A Physician's Guide to Therapeutic Massage* (second edition). Vancouver, B.C., Canada: Massage Therapists' Association of British Columbia. 1999.

Zemach-Bersin, David, Kaethe Zemach-Bersin, and Mark Reese. *Relaxercise.* New York: NY, HarperCollins Publishers. 1990.

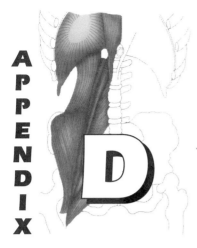

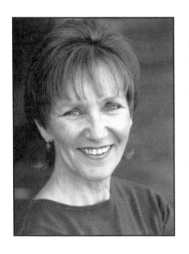

Carole Osborne-Sheets has been a private practitioner of integrative body therapies since 1974. Her focuses are understanding the connections between and releasing emotional and neuromuscular tensions. She is especially experienced in working with members of dysfunctional families and with childbearing, sexual and emotional abuse, self-image, and nurturing issues.

Her training includes study with the Arica Institute, the Yokefellow Center, the Trager, Upledger, and the Jones Institutes. She apprenticed in structural balancing with Edward Maupin, Ph.D., and studied extensively with tai chi master Abraham Liu and other tai chi teachers, and with Raymond J. Hruby, D.O.

In 1977, Carole co-founded the Institute of Psycho-Structural Balancing (IPSB), now the International Professional School of Bodywork, in San Diego where she continues to teach. She co-created and taught Bodywork for the Childbearing Year℠ for 14 years. She is the developer of and currently teaches Pre- and Perinatal Massage Therapy certificate workshops and other seminars throughout North America and Europe. She has published several articles, developed a variety of bodywork curricula and publications, and in 1998 completed her textbook, *Pre- and Perinatal Massage Therapy*. She is Nationally Certified in Therapeutic Massage and Bodywork.

She lives near San Diego, California, with her husband and two children.

Body Therapy Associates

9449 Balboa Avenue Ste. 310 • San Diego, CA 92123
Phone: 800.586.8322 • Fax 858.277.8827 • www.bodytherapyassociates.com
Visit our secure website for on-line orders and class registrations.

PUBLICATIONS AND VIDEOS

		Quantity	Cost
$28.95	***Deep Tissue Sculpting*** **(Second Edition)**	_____	$_____

Theory and practice of deep tissue massage for release of chronic myofascial tension; detailed instructions, photos, and guidelines.

		Quantity	Cost
$44.95	***Pre- and Perinatal Massage Therapy 2nd Edition*** explores massage	_____	$_____

and bodywork that enables massage therapists to support mothers and their babies throughout the childbearing year. In this updated edition, three technique manuals teach clinically refined and fully illustrated techniques. Thoroughly updated, reflecting the latest research findings and practices its four new chapters expand upon such critical topics as gestational complications, positioning, ethics, and business considerations. It includes new techniques, enhanced by online video segments of these used in the context of five sessions, and more. (See detailed description online at www.bodytherapyassociates.com)

		Quantity	Cost
$10.00	***Massage Therapy and Movement for Infants***	_____	$_____

Techniques and resources specifically for therapists' infant clients.

		Quantity	Cost
$19.95	***Tai Chi for Health*** **DVD**	_____	$_____

Improve tableside body mechanics with beginning instruction in Yang style tai chi. (2 hrs.)

		Quantity	Cost
$199.00	***Side Lying Positioning System***	_____	$_____

Designed by Carole Osborne, in collaboration with Oakworks, this system is the ultimate in comfort for sidelying positioning, particularly for pregnant women.

CONTINUING EDUCATION

Rhythmic Deep Tissue (Blends) Introduction (14 hours)
Effective, nonintrusive integrative soft tissue techniques; Based on textbook, *Deep Tissue Sculpting*

Pre- and Perinatal Massage Therapy (32 hours)
Comprehensive certification training for pregnancy, labor, postpartum; Based on textbook, *Pre- and Perinatal Massage Therapy*

(Contact Body Therapy Associates for tuition cost, schedule, and registration.)

$95.95	**Prenatal Massage Therapy Safety Essentials**	_____	$_____

Seven hour home study course

	Subtotal	$_____
(CA residents add 8.75% sales tax)		$_____
Shipping and Handling: 0-30...$9.50; 31-48...$11.50; 49+ ...$13.50		$_____
	TOTAL ENCLOSED	$_____

Price and availability subject to change.
Please make credit card, check or money order payable to Body Therapy Associates.

Name _____ ❏ Order & payment included
Street _____ ❏ Send workshop information
City/State/Zip _____
Telephone _____ E-mail _____
❏ MC ❏ Visa _____ Expiration_____
Signature of cardholder _____

First Edition Comments...

In this compact, easy to handle book, Osborne-Sheets brings together a great deal of information usually available only in lectures at those massage schools that teach connected touch and at workshops.
— Reviewed in *Massage Therapy Journal*, Fall 1991

"This is not just a technical manual. It offers clear descriptions of the principles upon which soft tissue therapy is based."
— Raymond Hruby, D.O., Past-President of the American Academy of Osteopathy

"The real strength of this book is its artistic presentation. It offers a rare insight into the psyche of the massage practitioner who has transitioned into an artist...A must for anyone in the massage profession sincerely interested in becoming a professional and becoming an artist."
—Paul St. John, reviewed in *Massage* magazine

"The first technical manual from which a therapist can actually learn deep tissue massage… An excellent textbook by one of the finest teachers in the U.S."
—David Lauterstein, co-owner Lauterstein-Conway Massage School.

Second Edition Comments...

Carole's thoughtful attention in laying out expanded text and graphics for ease and depth of learning, give this new edition exceptional value as an instructional tool for both educators and students.
— Jennifer Hicks, co-founder and instructor, Big Sky Somatic Institute, Helena, MT

Carole Osborne-Sheets' conversational style invites bodyworkers, massage therapists and all other health care providers into the compelling healing modality of Deep Tissue Sculpting. Once, there, the author makes complex concepts accessible, capturing both the apprenticeship and rich oral traditions in education of the bodywork profession. The book and the modality itself are grounded firmly in the history of body-mind approaches, in careful references to medical science, and in Osborne-Sheets' own generous philosophy of healing. This philosophy is made concrete by including solid self-care principles for the therapist, fluid techniques, and clear listening skills. But on an even deeper level, it honors the uniqueness and dignity of each client and therapist. This Second Edition of Deep Tissue Sculpting is a well-researched, wonderfully crafted contribution to the field. It is a valuable text for students and experienced practitioners alike.
— Tracy Walton, Academic Dean, Muscular Therapy Institute, Cambridge, MA

I have used Deep Tissue Sculpting as a student, therapist, and teacher. As a student I found the First Edition informative and user friendly. Carole's writing style has a warm feel while being clear and to-the-point, and it is reminiscent of her presence in the classroom. The book offers specific protocols for three common client complaints, while offering insight and encouragement for modifying sessions to serve the individual client, which is valuable to both the student and the therapist. As a teacher and school owner, I have found the book well organized, and even better so in the Second Edition. It has served us well as our primary text for deep tissue work for as long as I have been teaching. I highly recommend Deep Tissue Sculpting to anyone who practices, teaches or is just interested in bodywork.
— Ron Floyd, co-founder and instructor, Big Sky Somatic Institute, Helena, MT

Thank you, Carole! As a teacher, I have found the Sculpting book to be an incredible treasure. Not only does it clearly instruct, on the level of technique, but it gives a deep and powerful sense of the intention and artistry behind the work. This book is an inspiration to both student and teacher, and a valuable guide to any therapist working through the connective tissue web.
— Diana Panara, M.S.W., H.H.P.; Instructor, IPSB, San Diego, CA

As always, the same thorough attention, care and sensitivity that Carole brings to her training workshops for therapists is evident in her writing. This second edition of Deep Tissue Sculpting is an important book for massage therapists who are looking for more effective yet gentle ways of working with fascia therapeutically in the context of the whole person.
— Linda Hickey, Registered Massage Therapist, Calgary, Alberta, Canada

Carole Osborne-Sheets' Deep Tissue Sculpting provides a rounded, well referenced, and easy-to-use introduction to the world of structural bodywork. Although hand-to-hand teaching is always the best way to learn any manual technique, Carole's careful presentations and clear graphics make this book a valuable addendum to classroom work. The beginner will find many new approaches to all parts of the myofascial body, and even the experienced practitioner can find moves he may have forgotten or missed in this valuable library of techniques. The Second Edition incorporates a decade's worth of corrections, clarifications, additions, and refinements. I recommend taking on the initial chapters of this book as a good general bedside read from an author who sets this clinically sound but artistic approach in a refreshingly inclusive, broad context. Let Deep Tissue Sculpting then come to rest on a shelf near your practice table so that the technique chapters can inform your daily work.
— Tom Myers, Director, Kinesis, Inc.; author of *Anatomy Trains*

This book is clear, precise, well written and based on years of the wisdom only gained by intelligent experience. Carole Osborne-Sheets is one of the innovative leaders in the body therapy field. If you work with the body, you should read her book.
— Ben Benjamin, Ph.D., Author of *Listen to Your Pain*; founder Muscular Therapy Institute, Cambridge, MA

Deep Tissue Sculpting is an inspiring and artistic piece of work. I particularly enjoyed the passion and respect for the body that is evident in each chapter.
— Liz Ellis, massage therapist, Chicago, IL

Carole Osborne-Sheets writes with a clear voice of experience: as an educator, a clinician, and as an author. Mrs. Osborne-Sheets crafts words into a refined tool to take the reader deeply into the body of her knowledge. She educates the reader to penetrate skillfully and deeply into the body and mind of their client. The text is clear, direct, and practical with excellent illustrations that enhance and enrich the text.
— Rick Gold, author *Thai Massage: a Traditional Medical Technique*

Carole Osborne-Sheets is one of the premiere bodyworkers, and her presentation of deep tissue touch guides the student gracefully and well. But more than that, her personal compassion and sensitivity are always in the background, where intuition exceeds technique, and genuine substance underlies the outer form.
— Ed Maupin, Ph.D., Rolfer, structural balancing instructor, IPSB, San Diego, CA